Conflicts of Care

Award Recipient of the IMEW trainee's award for an outstanding scientific work

Helen Kohlen is junior professor for care policy, ethics, and community nursing at the Theological-Philosophical University of Vallendar, Germany.

Helen Kohlen

Conflicts of Care

Hospital Ethics Committees in the USA and Germany

Campus Verlag
Frankfurt/New York

Editorial Memo:
For all detailed interviews and participant observations, please refer to
www.campus.de/isbn/9783593388144

Bibliographic Information published by the Deutsche Nationalbibliothek.
Die Deutsche Nationalbibliothek lists this publication in the Deutsche Nationalbibliografie;
detailed bibliographic data are available in the Internet at http://dnb.d-nb.de.
ISBN 978-3-593-38814-4

For further information:
www.campus.de
www.press.uchicago.edu

Contents

Relational Analysis
Care and Hospital Ethics Committees

Practical Arena Analysis
Practices in Hospital Ethics Committees in Germany

Acknowledgement

I would like to thank the *Hanns Lilje Foundation* in Hannover for the doctoral scholarship that allowed me to concentrate on the dissertation full-time for two years. I am also grateful to the *Frauenförderprogramm* of the University of Hannover that funded six months to finish the dissertation. Moreover, the Lilje Foundation was helpful to finance two stays in the USA as a visiting scholar and supported the publication.

In July 2004, the Center for Bioethics at the University of Minnesota offered me a wonderful chance not only to do my independent research on the history of bioethics, but the faculty and secretary women (especially Karen Howard) were very helpful to arrange interviews and meetings that could help to follow my research questions. I thank the director, Jeffrey Khan, for "making everything possible". I also want to thank the co-director, Dianne Bartels, who spent more than once her time to inform me about the local history of Hospital Ethics Committees and I thank Deborah de Bruin who supported me in bringing forward my ideas about Bioethics. This stay I can now see as a key point of the research process would never have happened without Joan Liaschenko. From the beginning to the end of my work at the center, the time I spent with her was exceptionally rewarding academically as well as personally. In 2005, I spent a fruitful time at the Massachusetts General Hospital in Boston and at the Center for Health Policy and Ethics in Omaha, Nebraska. I thank Ruth Purtillo and Ellen Robinson, Pamela Imperato, Hanns de Ruyter, Leslie Kuhnel and Mary Faith Marshall for very rich interviews and I especially thank the director of the center, Amy Haddad, for sharing ideas, arrange meetings and for having spare-time together.

Whenever I felt lost or irritated during this research journey I knew where to go: The colleagues and friends of the doctoral colloquium, Isabella Jordan, Svea Luisa Hermann, Sabine Könninger, Torben Klussmann, Marion Schumann and Elke Wohlfart, supported me through all the steps of the dissertation. I especially like to remember sitting together and organizing the empirical data in the middle of the analytic process. At a certain step of data collection, Christel Conzen, Gudrun Woscholski, Marianne Rabe and Rosemarie Kerkow-Weil were also helpful to structure the empirical findings.

I wish to thank all the participants and members of the ethics committees as well as the hospital physicians and nurses who did not hesitate once to spend their time for an interview.

I could certainly not have better supervisors than Kathrin Braun and Barbara Duden. While Kathrin knew exactly how to handle and answer my questions in a specific balance of support and giving me the feeling of independence, Barbara would never stop challenging ideas that could turn everything upside down.

To finish the work, Andrea Wernecke, Birgit Schwillow and Natascha Riedel helped with refinements and language corrections. For the final (native speaker) language revision I thank Jan Marie Lützen. Rüdiger Otte could always find a solution for problems with regard to the typesetting. I also thank him for his patience that was needed for the layout and all preparations of the print. I am grateful to Heiko Geiling who made it possible to have an office at the Department of Political Science at the University of Hannover to write the dissertation. Stefan Meise and Dennis Eversberg were good company to have around next door, not only for coffee breaks, but also for lively academic talks.

Finally, I want to thank my daughters, Alice and June for all their humour while watching me – too often – either reading or writing. I thank their grandparents for spending holiday times with their granddaughters. My husband, Thomas Schwarzer has been involved in manifold most encouraging and pragmatic ways to start the dissertation, and keep developing my own ideas. I would enjoy giving it back.

Introduction

Problem Statement and Research Question

What is the use of Hospital Ethics Committees? Who do they serve? Who gets a voice and who does not get the time and authority to tell what the "real conflicts" are, for example, of a patient, the family or the medical and nursing team. What are the conditions that create problems of and around dying in a hospital? How does a committee actually work behind closed doors? Who demands to have the power of defining what an "ethical" problem is?

These are questions that do not only arise when analyzing empirical data of this work, like the dialogue presented above, but they have also been evolving by exploring the phenomenon of Hospital Ethics Committees within the context of bioethics. Nevertheless, by thinking about these questions and observing Hospital Ethics Committees' discursive practices in Germany, my focus at some point shifted from what is talked about to the unsaid and invisible. Hereby, questions of and around care practices evolved. Like any professional practice, care practices are generally understood as a coherent and complex set of activities with standards of excellence that help to make practice what it is and cannot be fully understood apart from it. Each practice is lived out in a specific way, and influenced in conditions of structural change like health care reforms.

The tradition of medicine has until now been characterized by an aspiration to provide as complete as possible a service of care for the populations for which it had responsibility. The same accounts for nursing and caring practices, but the tradition is loosening. Despite the collective assumption that medical and nursing practice rests on solid grounds of knowledge and a caring ethos, changes of practices have not only come about in a complex and diffuse fashion, but also come along with sacrifices, losses and deficits.

Managed care, invented and developed in the USA, recently implemented in Germany, provides one example that is promising efficiencies by eliminating assumed "wasteful" and "unnecessary" care. Managed care is an example, reminding that the doctor-patient-relationship as well as the nurse-patient-relationship does not take place as an isolated dyad, but is strongly influenced by its institutional and economic context. What US-American medical sociologists like Charles Bosk and Joel Frader (1998: 94) once commented on for the situation in the USA can now be said for changing processes in German Health Care.

The growth of ethics committees is another new phenomenon in Germany. Ethics committees were created in the USA not only in order to discuss ethical research questions, but also problems in clinical care. In the USA as well as in Germany, the need for ethics consultation and the building up of committees is generally explained by referring to technical progress that had changed Health Care. I will argue, whether and how these changes in medical research and clinical work, cannot simply be explained by technical progress, but possibly by reactions to external economic and socio-political forces as well as to ethical manoeuvres themselves. For the historical analysis my questions are: What were the forces and conditions that drove the increasing numbers of Hospital Ethics Committees? And, what were the manoeuvres for the discursive practices of these committees?

Situating the Field of Analysis and Approaching the Subject Matter

In the past, the community and neighbourhood, also the church, gave comfort and help to someone in need. Problems such as solitude, despair, or fear to go on living were dealt with on a direct communal basis. These rather *informal arrangements* are almost or not completely substituted by an expanding network of health care institutions and formal settings to offer consultations. Health care services are increasing in number and also the role of health care professionals is becoming more important. These specialized and institutionalized organizational forms are called the professional care sector or *care market*. Nursing, understood as a differentiated system of specialized nurses, practices, nursing institutions and nursing science is a part to secure health care.

Not saying this is a good or a bad thing, despite a long exile in the private domain, caring is becoming a subject of public discourse. It is remarkable, that currently in various fields of political debate, like education, family, or labor politics, an international care-debate has found its attention.[1] One example that care is becoming a political concern in Germany is shown by the current debate on a change of care-arrangements for children, and whether it can be justified that East European women do nursing care at home for the old, ill, and disabled people, earning two Euros for an hour of care work. The minister, who has gone about new governmental regulations in child care has also announced to put policy questions around elderly care on the agenda.[2] The political debate about care shows the prevailing ambivalence that a matter of concern that once belonged to the private domain is now turning into an affair of the state. The work of care falls outside of the field of productive activity and carries the problem of how its worth could ever be expressed in economic terms.

In Germany, along the process of health care *reforming,* modern bioethics as a discipline as well as a practice has become established within the last fifteen years. With regard to burning issues, one impulse for the evolution of applied ethics in German Health Care arose from a widely spread discourse on reproductive technology, gene-therapy, and embryo research.[3] Moreover, care at the end of life and Euthanasia have been incessantly crucial issues of the bioethical discourse in Germany. Since 2004 questions about end-of-life care at the bedside have for the first time been becoming a dominant point of issue by *governmental committees:* Questions in the framework of patients' autonomy, the use of Living Wills and Withholding and Withdrawal of Treatment have become a policy issue for the *Enquete Commission on Ethics and Law in Modern Medicine of the German Bundestag,* for the *National Ethics Council* as well as for a working group established by the *Federal Ministry of Justice*[4] in Germany. Their published drafts for legislation show different positions, revisions were made, but it has not come to an agreement yet.

I would like to point to what is new about these handlings. The fact that currently in Germany difficult end-of-life questions are answered by a demand for written forms of Living Wills to secure patients' autonomy is one remarkable change in medical and nursing practice. Furthermore, the fact

1 As exemplified in the work by Birgit Pfau-Effinger und Birgit Geissler (ed.) (2005): *Care and Social Integration in European Societies.*
2 An example for this current political debate is the "Aktionsprogramm für Mehrgenerationenhäuser" (2005–2007) of the "Bundesfamilienministerium" (BMFSJ).
3 See for example the issues presented in the book *Bioethik. Eine Einführung,* edited by Marcus Düwell and Klaus Steigleder in 2003.
4 See: Bundesministerium der Justiz (BMJ) (2004). See also Volker Lipp (2005) who comments on the debate from a juridical perspective.

that the debate on the use of Living Wills has now prompted governmental intervention is another significant turning point since caring practices at the bedside have never been regulated by political authorities before.

On a micro-political level, the new regulations are discussed by local ethics forums, termed Institutional Ethics Committees (IECs), Clinical Ethics Committees (CECs) or Hospital Ethics Committees (HECs) as they have once been invented in the US in the 1970s. Ethics committees were created in the US not only in order to discuss ethical research questions, but also problems in clinical care. Besides taking responsibility for staying informed on major bioethical issues with clinical relevance like regulations of Living Wills, Hospital Ethics Committees serve to develop, review, and apply the ethics policies or guidelines in and of the institution. In US-American hospitals, the most common form of ethics policy is the "Do Not Resuscitate" (DNR) policy, which sets out the institution's guidelines for withholding or withdrawing life-sustaining treatment. Moreover, Hospital Ethics Committees are responsible for case review. The kind of review varies. The committee can be directly involved in prospective case review and becomes a consultant to assist in the ongoing management of care of patients. Committees do usually also offer retrospective case review. Then, the goal is to determine whether and how the case could have been better dealt with. In addition, these committees play an educational role. Education involves mediation techniques and learning theoretical frameworks as well as the training to use a special "model of ethical decision-making" in order to discuss an ethical issue reasonably. With regard to actors, such committees consist of small groups of people, professionals as well as lay persons, who meet on a regular basis to address so called "ethical" issues that emerge within the health care institution. Those people are mainly clinical professionals, like physicians, nurses, chaplains, and social workers. Among them, there is sometimes a lawyer and, at least one person who is in the position of being an "ethics expert", usually a philosopher or a theologian. The group is acting behind closed doors at a certain place and time, and may serve themselves, the patient, relatives of the patients, a special unit, or the entire hospital.

The number of Hospital Ethics Committees has especially been increasing since the German Accreditation Organizations of Health Care have demanded that hospitals should have policies and procedures to cope with ethical issues. The rapid growth of ethics committees is a new phenomenon in Germany and qualitative research what the actors of and in these committees are actually doing, is missing.

The establishment of Hospital Ethics Committees demands that there is a *room for reflection* – in a denotative as well as in a figurative sense – within the hospital setting. This is unusual for daily clinical work since nursing as well as medical practice is action-orientated. The criteria of urgency shapes the communication culture, not the play on elaborate words based on theoretical frameworks. Dealing with critical situations of ill or dying patients is part of the everyday practice of nurses and medical doctors. An interdisciplinary ethical consultation while sitting around a table – away from the patients' bedside – is in some way odd since it implies the transformation of an original non-verbal act, highly shaped by sensitive competencies, into a discursive matter of fact. Therefore, Hospital Ethics Committees represent a *new type* of coping with conflicts in clinical practice as well as a new way of consultation and participation.

Purpose and Significance of the Study

The aim of this work is to understand the phenomenon of bioethics by committee practices in the hospital setting. Hospital Ethics Committees are the locus of this investigation which is not primarily concerned about bioethics as a discipline, but about its effects *in* and *on* medical and nursing practice. Hospital Ethics Committees are seen as a suitable institutional field to analyze a new type of coping with conflicts in clinical practice as well as a new type of consultation and participation practices. I will use these committees as a vehicle to shed light on a part of the process-transformations in clinical practices and the way caring issues are dealt with. Since caring practices are mainly carried out by nurses they are the actors mostly of interest here.

Moreover, nurses are by far the biggest group of professional health care, especially in the hospital. The World Health Organization assigns nurses and midwives to have a decisive role in Europe with regard to the development of strategies in health care reforms. Reforms in health care that demand high standards on quality, efficiency and a humanistic ethics at the same time, need to consider the participation of nurses. Nurses – even though not many – do participate within the academic discourse. Nevertheless, care work and those who mostly fulfill caring practices are usually unseen and undervalued. Nursing matters have mostly been invisible on the political agenda of German Health Care. Although nursing has become an academic discipline within the last 20 years in Germany, its lobby is weak in comparison to the medical profession. They are still struggling for more political power, institutionally as well as academically.

Nurses have hardly expressed their own position on bioethical issues within their academic discipline and do rarely show up within the public debate. Even though decisions will have a strong impact on their practice, nurses hardly raise their voice, and are even less listened to. In keeping its development as an academic discipline, nurses want to transform their knowledge from a record of experiences to a logical organization of relevant knowledge.

Within the last 15 years, US-American and Canadian nursing scholars, especially Joan Liaschenko (1993a, b) and Patricia Rodney (1997) have investigated the ethical concerns of practicing nurses and noted in their separate empirical research the invisibility of their conflicts when doing care work. Do these conflicts and concerns find a place in Hospital Ethics Committees?

From a political science perspective, studying professions can open a crucial dimension of the intermediary realm between individual and state. Professions are political entities, not just when they form interest groups, but because in the intermediary realm of civil society, professions possess the power to distract, encourage, limit, and inform public recognition of as well as deliberation over social conflicts. For reasons pointed out above, nurses are a suitable group to investigate into unknown spaces of Hospital Ethics Committees' practices, to question the definition of what counts as an "ethical" problem and who dominates the committee discussions. Moreover, the focus on nursing helps to shed light on different voices and can bring questions of care to a head.

Development of the Research Process and Structuring

The work is structured into four parts. While the first part situates the work in social science research, theoretically and methodologically, the following three parts build the corpus of analysis.

The structure of three analytical parts gradually developed during the research process. The original thesis of this project was that the hierarchical and increasingly economically orientated principles of hospitals, influence the demanded democratic procedures of ethics consultation and Hospital Ethics Committees. Hereby, the participation of the nursing profession might be impeded in a particular way and the conflicts they experience could be excluded. If a group who delivers the biggest amount of direct care is not participating in defining, discussing and resolving what the "ethical" conflicts of daily patient care are, then the search for an argumentation would be in need.

By an international literature review and expert interviews in the US, the phenomenon of Hospital Ethics Committees was approached by a broader social science perspective that included an inquiry of the historical background of these committees. I identified surprising silences in the discourse of Hospital Ethics Committees and had to refine my research questions. Finally, the research process combines three areas: Hospital Ethics Committees, the development of bioethics and care. How was this triangulation brought out?

The decision of exploring the historical background of contemporary Hospital Ethics Committees lead me to the origins and development of bioethics as an influential force that has shaped the work of these committees. The identification of the forces and the analysis of the way questions and issues were constructed in the development of US-American Hospital Ethics Committees revealed what has been becoming at stake, what and who is sidelined, transformed or ignored for whose and what interest (Historical Analysis).

One of the silences I identified in the bioethics discourse concerned questions of care and more specifically caring issues and conflicts. Why care matters, why and how it needs to be seen as something being of relevance, and more specifically, what international empirical literature tells about the work of Hospital Ethics Committees, issues of care and nurses' participation became the following theoretical part of the analysis (Relational Analysis).

Consequently, the study of what has been present and implicated in the history of Hospital Ethics Committees as well as what has *not* been present and implicated (conflicts of care), sharpened my ears and eyes for the participant observations and interviews in the practical arena. The field research was carried out as a parallel process of the theoretical analysis over two years in three Hospital Ethics Committees in Germany (Practical Arena Analysis).

How did the chapters of each part evolve?

The *Historical Analysis of Bioethics and Hospital Ethics Committees* is shaped by the following findings that emerged in the literature review and interviews: The more I read about ethics committees and the more I talked to people who declared themselves to be part of the history of bioethics as the interviews in the US show, the more colorful the picture became. Most authors start with the bright side of ethics committees seeing it as a helpful instrument to meet "moral insecurity" due to technological progress and a plurality of values. And this, they state, does not only account for professionals at the bedside, but also among people in public. Especially proponents of Hospital Ethics Committees do usually not write about the precursors to modern ethics committees. But as I found out, the history is surprisingly rich to show that consultation by committees can be reconstructed as a sequence of different sorts of problems and events.

Hospital Ethics Committees are identified as a part of the development of bioethics. By foregrounding the evolution and the style of bioethics, its move into the practical arena of hospitals is described in the first chapter. Then, traces and beginnings of consultation by committees will be presented. The rise of research ethics committees and the forms of governmental intervention will be included in the second chapter. In chapter three, the history of contemporary Hospital Ethics Committees will be traced back by starting with the story of Karen Quinlan. Since it is the United States where Hospital Ethics Committees were first invented, German literature mostly refers to US-American committee models, and even looks back historically by re-telling the "Quinlan case". As said in the introduction, social science research on these committees is missing. For these reasons of analysis, a description of the German development of Hospital Ethics Committees comes short at the end of the historical part. The historical analysis is summed up in the end (chapter four).

The following considerations and questions are relevant for the turn to *Care and Hospital Ethics Committees in the Relational Analysis:* What are the reasons why caring issues have never been at the forefront of bioethical debates, especially on a political level? First, an overriding as well as convincing argument for this marginalization is seen in the protection of keeping care as a private activity. Second, it is common sense, that caring is something practical that simply needs to be done and that there should be a kind of obligation to integrate caring within one's daily activities. Thus: Why theorizing about a daily private activity? However, there are also plausible reasons to defend a public debate on care since care work has been more and more institutionalized over the last century, at least in Western societies. Especially for a growing number of the elderly the need for care is increasing. While media reports on (health) care tend to focus on the high costs of the health care system, other dimensions and aspects of social service can get easily played down. The quality of care practices are of rare interest except when care has gone wrong, is done badly, or has even led to abuse. Then, public attention is aroused.

The aim of this part is to approach a refined understanding of care that lays out a language to describe the meaning of care and caring practices. These theoretical approaches are all written in a remarkable non-technical language, but unfortunately, some, especially the nursing ones, lack some clarity. Nevertheless, what I am not going to do is what Doris Lessing has once warned against in her *Golden Notebook* (1972), is: to criticize the criticism of ideas. I will neither atomise and belittle the weak parts of the concepts of care, although, of course, I will sum up the main critique that was put forward against them.

In the first chapter, I present the transitions of the care ethics debate since the 1980s when professional nursing care expanded. The chapter gives an overview to understand concepts of care within their specific contexts of ethical debates. Chapter two presents those ideas that have contributed to develop an understanding of care as a practice from a feminist as well as a political perspective. By referring mainly to the theoretical approaches by Joan Tronto, Elisabeth Conradi and Margaret Urban Walker, I want to contribute to the development of a language that realizes concerns regarding issues of care in medical and especially nursing practice. In chapter three, concerns of care in hospital nursing practice will be analysed and nurses' chances of making them a subject of discussion in Hospital Ethics Committees will then be outlined. While chapter one and chapter two are based on a literature review of mostly foundational texts from the US and Germany, chapter three will also make use of interviews (see Appendix)[5]. In the end, I will give a summary (chapter four) by focusing on those findings that are mostly relevant for the practical arena analysis, the empirical part.

The *Practical Arena Analysis* of three Hospital Ethics Committees in Germany took place from 2004 to 2006. In the field study, I examined the process of establishing a Hospital Ethics Committee by participant observations and interviews. In chapter one, the field research is introduced. A description will be given of how the methodological design, presented in the beginning, is specifically applied for the analysis of the practical arena. Then, each committee case story and their organizational structure will be outlined.

In the second chapter, the analysis of the field data that I collected out of twenty-three participant observations in the Hospital Ethics Committees and interviews, is presented. The look inside the committees has revealed

---

5 For all detailed interviews and participant observations, please refer to: www.campus.de /isbn/9783593388144

diverse practices with regard to the committee functions of education and policy making that I will show first. Then, I will turn to an analysis of the case discussions and evolving issues of concern. Finally, the analysis of the practical arena will be summarized. The *Appendix* contains the complete transcripts of the participant observations that I will refer to in the analysis by indicating the fictive names of the field subjects who talk and give reference signs. In the end (chapter three), I will discuss the findings of the practical arena analysis in connection with the findings of part one and two and then the conclusion will be drawn.

State of the Art, Theoretical Framework and Methodological Considerations

1 State of the Art in Social Science Research

Hospital Ethics Committees in Germany have neither been examined by foregrounding bioethics, nor in relation to caring and nursing. In 1998 the US-American sociologists Charles Bosk and Joel Frader published an article they called *Institutional Ethics Committees: Sociological Oxymeron, Empirical Black Box*. Bosk and Frader reflect the emergence and purpose of such forums by asking for more qualitative research that needs to be done (Bosk, Frader 1998). This accounts for the current situation in Germany.

Hospital Ethics Committees in Germany appear to be unknown discursive spaces behind closed doors. Published research has been limited to surveys which mostly provide quantitative data, e.g. about the numbers of committees that have been established.

The first clinical ethics committees were established in 1997. The German Lutheran and Catholic Church Association published a brochure that encouraged and called up to establish clinical ethics committees according to the US-American model. In 2000 a survey revealed that among 795 members of the Christian churches' association, 30 hospitals declared to have an ethics committee or a comparable arrangement to offer consultation.

A recent survey (Dörries, Hespe-Jungesblut 2007) shows that most of the German hospitals that have been established, or are in the process of building up, any kind of ethics consultation service, have decided for Hospital Ethics Committees. Most of the hospitals felt that they should have a committee in order to become certified by agencies that audit the quality standards of health care institutions. According to the survey, especially Lutheran and Catholic hospitals were motivated to build up a committee due to impulses given by the Christian Association of Hospitals. Hospitals also thought that an ethics committee could be an answer to a concrete ethical conflict they have currently been coping with. Finally, ethics committees were built up because the staff wanted it.

Like this publication, articles on Hospital Ethics Committees are written by philosophers, physicians, and sometimes theologians and biologists (Simon, 2000; Neitzke 2002, 2003; May 2004; Vollmann, Wernstedt 2005; Dörries 2007).

Unfortunately, at the time of writing, findings of the research projects on Hospital Ethics Committees in social science have not been published yet. The department of sociology of the Ludwig-Maximilian University in Munich in cooperation with the Lutheran-theological department of the University in Göttingen have been working on an interdisciplinary research project on organizational forms of Hospital Ethics Committees, and the department of Cultural Studies in Essen worked on a research project called *Clinical Ethics Committees, its Organizational Forms and Moral demands in Theory and Practice.*[6]

US-American social science publications explicitly on Hospital Ethics Committees are limited. Daniel Chambliss (1996) observed during his ten years of hospital field study that first, Hospital Ethics Committees tended over time to become somewhat dominated by legal, rather than ethical issues, and second, that these committees only enter the discussion after the health professionals at the bedside cannot or don't want to make a decision themselves, or the family disagrees with the professionals.

The research that my study can mostly relate to in its whole composition, is the dissertation by Patricia Flynn of the University of California, San Francisco, advised by Adele Clarke, called *Moral ordering and the social construction of bioethics* (1991a). She examined the emergence of the discipline of bioethics and its move into Hospital Ethics Committees as well as into a larger policy arena: community based bioethics committees. Flynn found that the disciplinary emergence of bioethics was an attempt to deal with developing problems of justice, and that decision-making processes in ethics both, at the policy level and at the local committee level (like Hospital Ethics Committees) are based upon a process of what she identified as "moral ordering". She defines rather generally:

---

6 Both projects were named at a conference I attended in Essen in 2002. Matthias Kettner and Arnd May wrote about the conference in a short report (2002), which however does not include findings.

"Moral ordering in health care is but one part of a broader moral ordering processes. [...] In bioethics today there is no [...] fixed moral order but instead a moral ordering and re-ordering about who is a person, what is an acceptable or unacceptable quality of life, how is death defined, and when shall we withhold or withdraw treatment. Many of these decisions are clearly social and ethical and not exclusively medical ones" (1991b: 146).

For the most part, however, Flynn argues that bioethical knowledge has been produced and re-produced in the image of medicine, and the medical profession has protected an incursion by law, ethics and government into their realm by "extending its own boundaries to include these other factions now reframed in medical terms [...] While government has attempted to define the boundaries of medicine's practice [...] , the medical profession has been successful at reclaiming its authority" (1991b: 155). Her study reveals that medicine absorbed the language of ethics and law, even transformed their principles into a new vocabulary and process used in committees. Thus, Flynn concludes that ultimately *biomedicine* defines the terms of the work of bioethics. "Having a committee to discuss bioethical issues implies that ethical issues will be discussed. [...] In fact, this is not true. The advice requested, and decisions made, are framed in terms of medicine and not ethics" (Flynn 1991a: 182). She also observed that in committee discussions there is much that is simply not picked up "[...] much that is cut off, many questions and interruptions [...] [since the] [...] medical discourse often cuts off contextual issues and redirects the focus to technical concerns. But it is not just physicians who do this. All who are using the medical discourse do so" (Flynn 1991a: 185).

2 Theoretical Framework and Research Design

New and unstudied research areas like Hospital Ethics Committees in Germany first demand exploration to approach the phenomenon. Not the testing of formal theories, but the development of theories, grounded in empirical data of cultural description is recommended for such new fields of social science research (Mayring 2002: 105–107).

When the methodological considerations unfolded during the research process in 2005, Adele Clarke's work *Situational Analysis* was published and proved to be the adequate choice to meet the complexity of my research questions. In the prologue of her book, Clarke explains: "What I am ultimately grappling toward are approaches that can simultaneously address voice and discourse, texts and the consequential materialities and symbolism of the nonhuman, the dynamics of *historical* change, and last but far from least, power in both its more solid and fluid forms" (2005: xxiii; emphasis added). The framework of Situational Analysis is new in its way of combining historical and discourse analysis with empirical research of the subject matter.

With roots in Chicago sociology, symbolic interactionism and pragmatic approaches to philosophy, *Grounded Theory* was originally developed in the late 1960s in the surroundings of Barney G. Glaser and Anselm Strauss (1967). It offers an empirical approach to the study of social and political life through qualitative research and distinctive approaches to data analysis. The procedure involves the continuous development, refinement and connection of evolving concepts, constructs and hypotheses. Therefore data gathering and data analysis happen simultaneously. In the course of the research process a theoretical framework is generated step by step through modification. Grounded Theory has classically been applied in field research in which the researcher has been involved as a participant observer.

Compared to Glaser and Strauss (1967), Adele Clarke (2005) sees Grounded Theory as "[...] conceptually much broader – not only fully sociological but also as pertaining to meso / organizational / institutional concerns [...] and also relevant far beyond sociology" (Clarke 2005: 18). She profoundly disagrees with Glaser's understanding of context in which it has to emerge as a relevant category or as a theoretical code like all other categories in Grounded Theories respectively, that it cannot be assumed in advance. On the contrary, Clarke has predicted Situational Analysis on the analytic necessity of addressing "context". She also contradicts Glaser's position that the goal of Grounded Theory should be a-historical, a-cultural, and transcendent. With reference to Donna Haraway (1988) she points out that there is no meaningful voice emerging from nowhere (Clarke 2005: 18).

For Clarke, "Knowledges and knowledge productions are situated and non-innocent" (2005: 18). Clarke is interested in assuming and acknowledging the embodiment and situatedness of all knowledge producers, and she aims to make the broader situation of the phenomenon under research the analytic ground (Clarke 2005: 21). Thereby, the researcher can draw on *interviews* as well as on *historical,* and other discursive material, including data arising from *field research.* "Situational analysis allows researchers to draw together studies of discourse and agency, action and structure, image, text and context, history and the present moment – to analyze complex situations of inquiry broadly conceived" (Clarke 2005: xxii).

Situational analysis includes the *comparative method* as used in Grounded Theory. Glaser and Strauss explain, whenever a comparison is drawn, for example between countries or institutions like the hospital, the correctness of the early impression about one country or hospital needs to be validated by comparing it with the other one(s). Comparison cases are sought out and used by the researcher to provoke analysis (Glaser, Strauss 1967, 1974). Adele Clarke understands this comparative method in its broadest sense as a strategic method that can be applied to social unities of any size.

Taking *history* seriously is a another key feature that is integrated in situational analysis (Clarke 2005: 261). Clarke emphasizes that the social phenomenon under research has to be understood in its historical context to make better sense of a contemporary situation of interest (2005: 262–264) and remarks: "This is what I mean by 'historicizing' contemporary research as compared to doing 'full-on' history" (2005: 265).

Furthermore, following Clarke, the primary path of Situated Analysis around the post-modern turn is through Michel Foucault (Clarke 2005: 52). She takes up Foucault's central point about *practices* by quoting him:

"(A)s in my other earlier work, the target of analysis wasn't 'institutions', 'theories' or 'ideologies', but practices – with the aim of grasping the conditions which make these acceptable at a given moment; the hypotheses being that these types of practice are not just governed by institutions, prescribed by ideologies, guided by pragmatic circumstances – whatever role these elements may actually play – but possess up to a point their own specific regularities, logic, strategy, self-evidence and 'reason.' It is a question of analysing 'regime of practices' – being understood here as places where what is said and what is done, rules imposed and reasons given, the planned and the taken-for-granted meet and intersect" (Foucault cited in Clarke 2005: 53).

For Clarke, there are strong echoes between Foucault's "regime of practices" and Anselm Strauss's "negotiated ordering". While Foucault focuses on the ongoing "how", that is to say, the ways in which a regime of practices must be sustained through performance of those practices over time, Strauss's "negotiated ordering" focuses on the management of contingencies in those practices through strategic negotiations, but similarly assumes ongoing practices (Clarke 2005: 53).

Foucault's concept of "discursive practices" describes ways of practices which could, when historically analyzed, produce dominant discourses that can put together injunctions about particular ways of being in the world (Dreyfus, Rabinow 1983: 59). Dominant discourses are reinforced through institutional systems of law, the media, or medicine and so forth. For instance, institutions of medicine, care and the media can together produce extensive discourses on health and the responsibilities of citizens to pursue it.[7] "Discursive formations are [...] capable of and routinely contain contradictory discourses [...] It is *through* this containment that some stability is achieved – however temporary, elusive, or conditional" (Clarke 2005: 54). Moreover, a discourse is effected in disciplining practices that produce subjects and subjectivities through surveillance, and various (self-) technologies, ways of a proper order in producing ourselves as disciplined subjects (Foucault 1974, 1986, 1988). Both, individuals and collectivities are constituted by the development and dynamics of discourses and disciplining (Foucault 1988). Clarke explains:

---

7 An example is demonstrated in an essay by Margaret Urban Walker (2006): The Curious Case of Care and Restorative Justice in the US Context.

"For Strauss, both individuals and collectivities are *produced* though their partici-pation in social world arenas, including their discourses. While Foucault's lan-guage of disciplining and the constitution of subjectivity(ies) is more insistent and decenters 'the knowing subject' much more thoroughly, these productions are ac-complished through routine practices. Later in his career, when issues of agency concerned him more, Foucault (1988:11; emphasis added) stated: 'I would say that if now I am interested, in fact, in the way in which the subject constitutes himself in an active fashion, by the practices of self, these practices are nevertheless *not* something that the individual invents by himself. They are patterns that he finds in his culture and which are proposed, suggested and imposed on him by his culture, his society *and his social group*'" (Clarke 2005: 57).

By the concept of 'situation' and the framework of Situational Analysis, Clarke seeks to capture these points outlined above, the situation qua con-ditions of possibility and the action, discourses, as well as practices in it. "I conclude by asserting that a worthy project, and part of doing situational analysis, is to learn how to productively take back and forth among these useful and provocative concepts analytically" (Clarke 2005: 59).

Adele Clarke suggests writing memos and designing maps as analyti-cally walking around, through and across the "social worlds / arenas" of investigation and "staring relentlessly until their commitments, ideologies / discourse, work organizations, technologies [...] can be specified" (Clarke 2005: 115). Similarly, the questions that should be raised are:

- "What is the focus of the arena?
- What social worlds are present and active?
- What social worlds are present and implicated or not present and impli-cated?
- Are there any worlds absent that you might have expected?
- What are the hot issues/contested topics/current controversies in the arena's discourses?
- Are there any surprising silences in the discourse?
- What else seems important about this arena?" (Clarke 2005: 115).

The "social worlds" that are identified as not being present in the arena, then become the next area of investigation, that is, following Clarke, the "relational analysis" (Clarke 2005: 102–108).

3 Method and Sources of Information

Germany and the United States:
Literature Review, Interviews and Pre-Study

For an overview about the local scene of Hospital Ethics Committees, the research was prepared by a literature analysis and informant interviews in Germany. The three-part analysis for understanding the emergence as well as the foundations of Hospital Ethics Committees demanded different ways and tools of gathering information and collecting data.

The first part is based on a US-American literature analysis of the history of Bioethics and Hospital Ethics Committees as well as expert interviews during a one month stay at the Center for Bioethics at the University of Minnesota in 2004 and a one week visit to the Center for Health Policy and Ethics at the University of Creighton (Omaha) in 2005. Moreover, there was given access to authentic institutional data of US-American hospitals and informants by visiting the Massachusetts General Hospital in Boston and the Alegent Health Care Hospital in Omaha in 2005. The second part of the study required an in-depth literature analysis on caring, nursing and committees. Interviews were also used as sources of information (see Appendix 1.1 and 1.2).

The third part consists of participant observations in three Hospital Ethics Committees in Germany over twenty months (October 2004 – July 2006), a Catholic Hospital in Southern Germany, a Lutheran Hospital in Northern Germany and a Municipal Hospital (then privatized) in Northern Germany as well. Before the main field research could start, a *pre-study* (survey) was needed to identify the hospitals that had started to build up an ethics committee nearly at the same time. This was done by attending conferences on Hospital Ethics Committees (University of Essen 2002, Academy of Tutzing in Munich 2003) and getting into contact with actors in the clinical field (door-openers).

Notes were taken from informative talks and interviews (see list of informant interviews in Appendix 1.1). The expert interviews were audio-taped and then transcribed (see list of expert interviews and transcripts in Appendix 1.2).

Field Research in Germany: Participant Observation and Interviews

Like in any qualitative orientated research, the method is specifically connected to the subject matter, and the instruments are specifically developed and differentiated for the research questions. An early definition of participant observation that focuses on the role of the observer refers to it as:

"A process in which the observer's presence in a social situation is maintained for the purpose of scientific investigation. The observer is in a face-to-face relationship with the observed, and, by participating with them in their natural life setting, he gathers data. Thus, the observer is part of the context being observed, and, by participating with them in their natural life setting, he gathers data" (Schwartz, Schwartz 1955: 344).

Reading definitions of participant observation since then (Becker 1958; Bruyn 1963; Mayntz, Holm, Hübner 1978; Spradley 1980; Lamnek 1995; Flick 1996; Mayring 2002), I found out that most of the characteristics are maintained that can be summed up as followed: In the first place, *participant observation* is not a single method but rather a characteristic style of research that blends a number of methods and techniques, like participant observations, informant interviewing, and content analysis as were combined in this study. Second, participant observation is intentionally unstructured in its research design in order to maximize discovery and description rather than systematic theory testing. That is, participant observers do not employ standardized concepts, measures, samples, and data, but rather seek to discover and revise these as they learn more about the organization being studied. Hence, analyzes and interpretation of data can present complicated problems of reliability, validity and comprehensiveness. Third, these anticipated problems are exacerbated by the fact that the resulting data are typically qualitative rather than quantified scores readily amenable for a standard statistical analysis. Fourth, participant observation is a relatively time taking and sometimes expensive procedure in that it demands not only months, but usually years of active field involvement for the researcher. Fifth, the practical problems met by the researcher have to be substantially lived through and require considerable thought and human relation work if months of effort are not to be distorted, jeopardized, or invalidated. One of the classical practical problems is the degree of the participant observer's involvement, both, *with* people and *in* the activities of the field being studied.

Theoretically, five types of participation are differentiated, arranged along the continuum of being a passive participant with low involvement, a moderate one with some involvement, an active one with high involvement, up to complete participation with the highest involvement.

Someone who has professional background experiences of the field, like the researcher here, could get into a role conflict by identifying too much with the actors in the field. Therefore, a moderate participation that seeks to maintain a balance between being an insider and an outsider, between participation and strict observation, proved to be the adequate choice to gain substantial data and still win the actor's trust. Nevertheless, the empirical part of this research fully demanded the work and strategies to keep the strengths of participant observation and to reduce its inherent weaknesses as much as possible.

Data Collection and Interpretation: Qualitative Content Analysis

The detailed written protocols of twenty-three participant observations of ethics committees' meetings served as the central empirical data being developed into the main material for the analysis. Narrative protocols and notes that were hand-written during the meeting were typewritten as soon after events as possible, routinely within twenty-four hours. Seventeen out of twenty-three were identified to be useful for the analysis (see Appendix 2.3 and 2.4).

In addition to the participant observations, twenty-eight informant interviews provided context-relevant as well as clarifying information that was needed to explicate and validate the observational data for interpretation. Moreover, subjective meanings for the participants could be identified and shed a different light on the preliminary findings. These persons, called informants, were not only the committee members, irregular participants, but also people of direct influence on the committee work as well as those whose relevance was shown by naming them in committee discussions.

Participant observation as well as expert and informant interviewing helped to provide a "thick description" (Geertz 1973) of the contexts given to the questions raised in the study. Clifford Geertz used this term for social inquiry that is both closely grounded in the data of fieldwork and imaginative in interpreting the connections and meanings found in the data (1973: 16). Adele Clarke states: "Thick analysis takes explicitly into account the full array of elements in the situation and explicate their interrelations" (2005: xxiii).

The collected data from the field research is approached by *Qualitative Content Analysis*. Three steps are followed for the interpretation: (1) *Summary*: The goal is to reduce the material in such a way that the dominant content elements are kept by creating an abstract corpus that can be overviewed and still depicts the basic material. (2) *Explication*: It aims to support individual text passages (notions, sentences) with adding materials which broadens the understanding, explains the text passage and interprets it. (3) *Structuring*: The purpose is to filter out certain aspects of the analysis based on ordering criteria that can take a cross-section through the material or to judge the material due to certain criteria.

The questions posed in the beginning of the field research were gradually refined within the analytical process and guided the choices of instruments. To make the logic of methods transparent, the actual field research will be documented in detail in Practical Arena Analysis. This refers to the explication of assumptions, combination of the instruments for the analysis, steps of implementation and gradual interpretation of the data.

Openness as well as a continuous structuring and re-structuring has marked the research process. The theoretical perspectives, methodological commitments, and method processes all engage cyclically with one another during the research. The quality of the interpretation was secured by a sequenced process of the analysis. All different steps were prepared ahead, but each one got its final shape within the actual research process. Going back and forth between the field data gathered from the participant observations and informant interviews, allowed comparing the findings. Although there could never be a total consent of the findings, the different perspectives could complement and correct each other.

Historical Analysis
Bioethics and Hospital Ethics Committees

1 US-American Bioethics and the Move into the Practical Arena

On a rather superficial level, what the people in the field call bioethics, is the study of "ethical issues" related to health sciences, such as the implications for the human well-being by innovations in health care as well as the use of human subjects in medical research. The term signals both an affiliation as well as a departure from the ancient discipline of medical ethics that is usually associated with the tradition of Hippocrates, centering on the internal problems of medical practice like the proper relations between physician and patient. Ethical codes of conduct are examples of what medical ethics deal with. Beyond serving professional interests, they govern qualities of care to directly benefit patients. While medical ethics is very much linked to professional obligation, bioethics is much more difficult to grasp with regard to its responsible actors and activities. This will be analyzed in the first part of this chapter before historical forerunners of Hospital Ethics Committees are laid out.

"Bioethics is not just Bioethics": Its Make and (Un)Concerns

Kathrin Braun (2000) has fundamentally been criticizing "bioethcis" and could reveal the gaps and traps of thinking and assuming that bioethics is "just" a new academic discipline. The statement "Bioethics is not just Bioethics" is borrowed from Renee Fox and Judith Swazey who used it as a headline for the conclusion of their article *Medical Morality is Not Bioethics – Medical Ethics in China and the United States* (1984). One goal of this published paper was to obtain a cultural perspective on what people in the United States term "bioethics". Fox and Swazey started to investigate into the phenomenon of bioethics by focusing on its cultural and historical contexts for expansion. The medical sociologist, Fox, has continuously been criticizing the movement of US-American bioethics. Her work is mostly of interest here. In the following, I will deal with the questions of *what* bioethics is understood to be, *when* and *why* it was understood to evolve and develop, and *who* the principal actors were. Moreover, I will take a look at its language style and framework.

"Bioethics": The Term and its Origins

Fox and Swazey (1984) criticize philosophers – explicitly Tristram Engelhardt – who has announced himself to be a "bioethicist" – for viewing bioethics as largely a-cultural and trans-cultural in nature. Later, Renee Fox explains in her article *More than Bioethics* (1996) that the expansionary use of the term ethics and bioethics is connected with a larger social phenomenon. For her, US-American bioethics is an expression and a part of the society and culture from which it has emerged. She argues:

"[...] bioethics is not, and never has been, 'just bioethics' [...] First, there has always been ambiguity about whether bioethics could or should be defined in strict disciplinary and academic terms. Although its founders and most prominent contributors have been highly trained in particular disciplines (pre-eminently philosophy, theology, the law, and medicine), from the outset of history, bioethics has been a multidisciplinary field, actively involved in clinical and policy application, as well as in reflection and inquiry, whose locus and outreach extend beyond the academy and professional enclaves into the public domain. Paradoxically, as bioethics has become more recognized and consolidated institutionally, the conception of the field, of its orbit, and of its practitioners has become more diffuse and imprecise" (Fox 1996: 6).

Fox observed that the term "bioethics" came into use in the US towards the end of the 1960s. For her and Swazey "Bioethics is the neologism coined in this country in the 1960s to refer to the rise of professional and public interest in moral, social, and religious issues connected with the 'new biology' and medicine and to the emergence of an interdisciplinary field of inquiry and action concerned with these issues" (Fox, Swazey 1984: 336).

To understand the flourishing of bioethics, Raymond DeVries and Peter Conrad are interested in the explanation of the profound public suspicion of medicine and the use of an ethical profession to respond to that suspicion. According to their analysis, three features were characteristic for the encouragement of bioethics in the United States: individualism, pluralism, secularisation.

"Because secularised society lacks a foundation for ethical decision making, moral dilemmas, once readily solved with reference to a faith tradition, now require the articulation of nonreligious solutions. Pluralism demands arbitration between cultures – a niche neatly filled by a bioethicist. And the rise of individualism [...] diminishes the role of community in ethical decision making, creating a need for ethical guidance" (DeVries, Conrad 1998: 240).

When did these three features of American society identified by DeVries and Conrad come together? DeVries and Conrad locate these characteristics historically back to the 1960s, when agitation over civil rights, the Vietnam war, and also the liberation of women led to widespread questioning of institutional authority and ambition to handle structural injustice. The authors remark: "The conduct of medicine did not escape scrutiny; the bioethics movement is the organized offspring of that scrutiny" (DeVries, Conrad 1998: 240). According to their analysis, the occupational world was then the one that supported the growing bioethical specialty (1998: 240). In the mind of an American, they suggest, the growth of knowledge is combined with the expectation of spawning new specialty areas. "More specifically, medicine, an occupation fragmented into many specialties, was [and is] organizationally prepared to accept an ethical specialist" (1998: 241). These forces and conditions prepared the ground for the development of bioethics they say.

Although modern bioethics as a discipline is mainly dated back to events of the 1960s when, for example, the kidney dialysis machine first came into service, there are a number of events earlier, that can certainly not be overlooked as an impact on its emergence.

The noise of the 1960s, Tina Stevens (2000) explains, has obscured the birth of bioethics and the fact that doctors and geneticists themselves first invited non-physicians to offer guidance. As physicians used resuscitation machines, they found themselves enmeshed in the process of prolonging the suffering of the dying. The International Congress of Anaesthesiologists sought help from Pope Pius XII, and a 1957 papal encyclical declared that stopping a resuscitation machine was acceptable if the purpose was to give an end to suffering (Stevens 2000). Some social scientists see the Nuremberg medical trials as a decisive historical landmark (Flynn 1991a, Wolpe 1998). Patricia Flynn argues:

"These trials bared contradictions between expectable medical practice and ethical standards of European and American culture. The trials themselves initiated wider negotiations about the medical moral order and were requisite for the construction of bioethics. The trials provided a first wedge of entree and allowed the incursion of the state into the internal dynamics of the medical world" (Flynn 1991a: 64).

What Counts as a Bioethical Problem?

The phenomenon with which bioethics is primarily concerned is usually related to problems associated with technological progress, and not to the promises they hold forth, like anticipated developments in genetic screening and counselling, birth technology, artificial kidney machines, life support systems, and organ transplantation. Bioethics has also been concerned with the proper definition of life and death as well as personhood. The justifiability of forgoing life-sustaining forms of medical therapy is another dominantly discussed concern in the clinical arena. One of the most evolving general characteristics of his ensemble of concerns is that they all cluster, at least to some degree, around problems of natality and mortality, that is to say at the beginning and at the end of human life. Another concern that has increasingly been emphasized since the mid-1970s is the allocation of scarce, expensive resources for advanced medical care, research and development. Fox and Swazey remark:

"The resources with which bioethics is chiefly concerned are material ones, mainly economic and technological in nature. The allocation of nonmaterial resources such as personnel, talent, skill, time, energy, caring, and compassion is rarely mentioned. Bioethics situates its allocation questions within a rather abstract, individual rights-oriented notion of the general or common good, assigning greater importance to equity than to equality. The ideally moral distribution of goods is defined as one that all rational, self-interested persons are willing to accept as just and fair, even if goods are allotted unequally" (Fox, Swazey 1984: 353).

Absent in bioethical deliberations about risk pools and Managed Care Organizations (MCOs) is a critique of the administrative costs of these organizations. "Bioethicists are busy determining formulas, recommending better informed consent for clients of MCOs, or finding ways to protect the physician-client relationship, but they are not asking if an MCO can ethically justify executive salaries over 1 million Dollar (before stock options) while denying a member proper instruction on breastfeeding after childbirth" (DeVries, Conrad 1998: 237). When Raymond DeVries and Peter Conrad write about the *The Blind Spots of Bioethics*, they point out that two questions, despite their importance, have not been considered yet: (1) "How does an issue get defined as bioethical?" (2) "Who speaks for bioethics?" (DeVries, Conrad 1998: 235).

Adam Hedgecoe wonders whether US-bioethicists have been silent on the topic of the ethics of healthcare funding and structure. He asks why inequitable access to healthcare and the lack of decent health provision for over 40 million people shouldn't be a topic of moral interest (Hedgecoe 2004: 126).

Technology as a Driving Force for Bioethics?

Coming back to the argument, generally found in bioethical literature, that new medical and technological advances drive bioethics to give answers to value questions, Raymond DeVries and Peter Conrad contradict: Although there is a simple elegance to this explanation, it is empirically false. The authors reflect that questions generated by new technology are not new. Although advances in technology have heightened ethical concerns in recent years, the issues of euthanasia, withholding or withdrawing treatment, truth telling, informed consent, as well as equitable access to health care have long been there, but "[...] they were just never on an open public agenda" (DeVries, Conrad 1998: 240). Moreover, the authors state, that technologies were not new to medicine. On the contrary, medicine had introduced new machines and new techniques regularly over the past century and many of them had reframed the moral questions of medicine. Partly due to its biomedical determinism, bioethical analysis usually ignores the fact that some of the same cultural questions that have been central to medical developments have also been central to many non-medical issues in American society.

As Raymond DeVries and Peter Conrad remark, the presence of technology did not necessarily call for a bioethical specialist. According to them, several existing occupations could have been asked, like lawyers, clergy people, and social workers who routinely advise in matters of life and death and were available to give counsel on the use of new technology in the 1960s and 1970s (DeVries, Conrad 1998: 240).

The Centrality of Individualism and the Principle of Autonomy

According to Fox, bioethics is not only a social and cultural, but also an intellectual happening. It has emerged within the growing culture of neo-individualism in the US-American cultural tradition and the emphasis on individual rights attached the value complex of individualism. Fox and Swazey are convinced that the emphasis bioethics places on individualism and contractual relations freely entered into by voluntarily consenting adults who would tend to minimize and obscure the interconnectedness of persons and the social and moral importance of their interrelatedness (Fox, Swazey 1984: 354). Although voices like Paul Ramsey's and Hans Jonas's were rare even then, but still venerated figures, it struck Fox that among bioethicists, their perspectives had little influence on the master conceptual framework of the field "[...] the principalism of analytic philosophy" (Fox 1996: 6). Fox and Swazey stress that the centrality of the principle of autonomy in Anglo-American analytic philosophy had been the regnant intellectual framework of American bioethical thought and state:

"[...] it is the individual, seen as an autonomous, self-determining entity rather than in relationship to significant others, that is the starting point and the foundation stone of American bioethics. Herein lie some of the deepest intellectual and philosophical difficulties that we have experienced as two of the relatively few social scientists who have been professionally associated with bioethics since its inception" (Fox, Swazey 1984: 339).

With regard to the 1980s, Fox talks about "[...] incipient changes in the ethos of American bioethics" (Fox 1990: 210). Critical commentaries by observers of bioethics as well as self-criticism[8] started to be discussed and were put forward. Fox observed that most philosophers-bioethicists contend that the triumph of the principle of autonomy had been essential for general moral and specifically medical reasons. After all, the key question of the criticism was not how to get rid of autonomy, but how to keep it from becoming such a moral focus and how to avoid that other values are ignored, "[...] particularly those that pertain to social ethical questions" (Fox 1990: 211). According to Renee Fox (1990), this concern was shown when the Hastings Center organized a symposium 'Autonomy, Paternalism, and Community' to celebrate its fifteenth anniversary in 1984: Caution was expressed with regard to an ethics based on maximizing individual autonomy while neglecting the obligation to the human community. Fox remarks:

"Central to all the symposium discussions was a preoccupation with the 'just allocation of scarce resources' [...] and with the fact that because of its strong individualistic focus, ethics had contributed relatively little to such large-scale, societal, health care delivery and policy issues. The statements made on this important rites-of-passage occasion seemed to presage greater future involvement of bioethics in what were termed 'large, structural, moral and political decisions'" (Fox 1990: 211).

---

8 For example, Daniel Callahan criticized too much emphasis on the language of rights of American individualism and of American courts (1980: 1230). In another article he points out that the principle of autonomy has been given an exaggerated importance whereas other values have not been sufficiently looked at (Callahan 1984: 42).

The Exclusion and Transformation of Social Matters

Fox resumes that the priority bioethics has accorded to individualism had not only diverted its gaze from particular kinds of social issues, in particular those that affect persons in society who are poor, discriminated against, and marginalized, but it had also drawn lines between what are defined as social and as ethical matters (Fox 1996: 7). Her most memorable example of the tendency of bioethics to separate the ethical and the social occurred during her service on the *President's Commission for the Study of Ethical Problems in Medicine and Biomedical and Behavioural Research* from 1979 to 1982. She recounts:

"[...] a number of commissioners argued that although inequitable access to health care in the United States was a serious problem, and we had been mandated by Congress to 'study the ethical and legal implications of differences in the availability of health services as determined by income or residence of the person receiving the service', it was not a topic appropriate for our deliberations because it was a social issue, with policy and political implications, rather than an ethical one. After a period of intense negotiation, the Commission agreed to undertake the study, and to include race and ethical origins as additional factors to be examined in evaluating differences in the availability of health care. The result was the volume entitled Securing Access to Health Care, published in March 1983, with whose conclusions not all the members of the commission agreed" (Fox 1996: 7).

Fox also observed that medical educators are presently inclined to affix the label "bioethics" to a good deal of what they try to teach medical students about the psychological, social, and cultural, as well as the moral aspects of health, illness, and medicine. And, she adds, that nowadays, a sociologist of medicine like herself is more likely to be introduced to whatever audience she addresses as an "ethicist" or "bioethicist", than a social scientist (Fox 1996: 6).

Bioethics has played a major role in framing its operational conception of what a "moral problem" is, in which religious, cultural, and social variables are not only sharply distinguished from moral, respectively ethical ones, but their relevance is minimized. As also Barbara Katz-Rothman observed, the overall orientation of theologians in bioethics is secular as well as un-sociological. When questions of a religious nature do arise in bioethics, there is a marked tendency either to screen them out or to reduce them in a way that they can be fitted into the field's circumscribed definition of ethics and what counts as ethical (Fox 1990: 208, Katz-Rothman 2001: 36–39).

Professional Participants and the Language of Bioethics

The term bioethics, like the field itself, was initially intended to represent a broad-based interdisciplinary field in which not only one discipline or discourse was to be dominant. The main intellectual actors and professional participants in American bioethics have been philosophers, theologians (pre-dominantly Catholic and Protestant), jurists, physicians, and biologists. This group was also followed by economists that became more relevant during the 1980s debate on the allocation of so-called "scarce resources" and when cost containment problems entered the field of bioethics. Moreover, public officials who have played a decisive role in the involvement of local and national government in bioethical matters have also influenced the outlook and emphasis of the field (Fox 1990: 205). Relatively few social scientists and nursing scientists have been actively involved or notably influential in bioethical debates, research, writing as well as action. And, although bioethicists have considered some political aspects of their field, such as macro-allocative problems like fair distribution of medical services, "the political nature of bioethics [...] is broader and deeper and cannot be reduced to such distributive issues [...] it shares in the power of the professional complex of medicine" as Albert Dzur remarks (2002: 178). According to Dzur, this context of institutional power raises issues of respresentation, consensus, coercion, publicity, and privacy (Dzur 2002: 178). Those issues that are rarely discussed in bioethical debates, have mainly been taken up by medical sociologists and anthropologists "to turn to democratic theory, especially deliberative democratic theory, to reconstruct their institutional practice" (Dzur 2002: 178). Fox and Swazey explain:

"The limited participation of anthropologists, sociologists, and political scientists in bioethics is a complex phenomenon, caused as much by the prevailing intellectual orientations and the weltanschauung of present-day American social science as by the framework of bioethics [...] the status and role of jurists in bioethics are integrally connected with the singular importance that Americans attach to the principle as well as to the fact of being 'a society under law, rather than under men'" (Fox, Swazey 1984: 350).

The authors think that the rationalism of American law, its emphasis on individual rights, and the ways in which it has been shaped by Western traditions of natural law, positivism, and utilitarianism, overlap with and reinforce the philosophical thought in bioethics. Fox points out that the cognitive and value traits of bioethics are a product of a number of converging factors. All in all, it is analytic philosophy "[...] with its emphasis on theory,

methodology, and technique, and its utilitarian, neo-Kantian, and 'contrac-
tarian' outlooks – in which the majority of the philosophers most active in
bioethics were trained" (Fox 1990: 208). Philosophical positivism is shaped
by the scientific principles and rules, of course, well-known by physicians
and biologists who have been educated and socialized to apply this style of
scientific thinking to their professional work. Enabling the courts and also
for the legislatures to make concrete decisions about the growing number
of bioethical cases, the problems are treated in a rather technical manner by
the application of legal principles. This means, for example, contextual concerns with regard to the 'definition of death' are transformed into statutory,
medico-legal criteria for pronouncing death, either on the basis of irrevers-
ible cessation of circulatory and respiratory functions. The courts turn to
the biological concept of "fetal life after viability", and to the legal concept
of 'right of personal privacy' (Fox 1990: 209).

Among professional participants of bioethics, a high value is placed on
logical reasoning – preferably placed on a general moral theory and concepts
derived from it. Rigor, precision, clarity, consistency as well as objectivity
are regarded as earmarks of the intellectually and ethically favourable kind
of moral thought. This way of thought tends toward dichotomous distinctions and bipolar choices as Fox and Swazey point out:

"Self versus others, body versus mind, individual versus group, public versus private, objective versus subjective, rational versus nonrational, lie versus truth, benefit versus harm, rights versus responsibilities, independence versus dependence,
autonomy versus paternalism, liberty versus justice are among the primary ones"
(1984: 355).

In addition to an analytical argumentation and a technical procedure in the
'grasping' process of ethical-problem definition and going into a decision-
making case, applied pragmatism is also influential. Applied pragmatism
contributes to the way bioethical problems are conceptualized and analyzed.
The actors, like physicians, nurses, hospital administrators, patients, families, lawyers, politicians, and their associates are expected to decide what to
do and what not to do in real-life (life-or/and death) settings, and then not
write or talk, but act on the ground of their determination and consensus
(Fox 1990: 209).

Since bioethicists are drawn from diverse professional groups, the proper
task of bioethics is not clear at all. Areas of study have their own vocabulary, and consequently, bioethics gets a conglomerated linguistic shape. The
language of bioethics tends to be specifically eclectic, because it has devel-

oped in an interdisciplinary setting and has gathered up the language from medicine, philosophy, theology, law, as well as ordinary life. Judith Andre remarks about the language of Bioethics: "We might think about this third language as a kind of pidgin, an analogy that can be developed in interesting ways. But little attention has been paid to this multilingualism, and as result we fall into some significant traps" (2002: 5). Barbara Katz-Rothman takes up John Evans's idea of "moral Esperanto" in the bioethical discussions:

"Esperanto was conceived as a shared language that a multitude of ethnic and linguistic groups would develop and use in the market. Like bioethics, it would be its own world with its own language, a neutral place where competing moral and ethical considerations could play out. But Evans shows that Esperanto is a language learned form the colonizers, and that in framing the problems, in expressing them in a particular language, certain solutions come to be seen as inevitable" (Katz-Rothman 2001: 36).

Because the issues of life and death convey strongly held values, the language bears a heavy emotional burden. The codification of moral values can have social effects since it frames debates in its own terms. As soon as an ethical vocabulary is adopted the following arguments have to fit into its terminology while the assumptions of the debate are controlled. Daniel Chambliss observed that the use of bioethical language has made moral debates more abstract by

"[...] continually referring to general principles [...], rights-driven, individualistic, and centered on discrete cases. Left aside, often, are discussions of the general routines or structures of medical services. Such language is legalistic in tone and sometimes indistinguishable from legal advice. An 'ethics consultation' in American hospitals often includes the hospital lawyer, and decisions on what is right are regularly tempered by what the courts officially sanction as legal. Where the language of ethics frames debate, certain issues find no place in the conversation. At the same time, this language can be a weapon for those who know it [...] this language was not created with nursing in mind, and the discipline of bioethics, recently expanded from medical ethics, has the most part bypassed nursing" (Chambliss 1996: 4).

The struggle to find a proper, mutually agreeable way of organizing themselves in order to gain legitimacy and strength has been more challenging for bioethicists than their effort to find a proper intellectual framework. It had taken bioethicists a decade-long of effort to develop standards for the profession, to establish a unified professional association that can speak for their subject matters, and to create a body of knowledge unique to the field (DeVries, Conrad 1998: 242).

What can be said at this point to resume how bioethics got its shape? There have been different opinions about the origins of the field as there have been different understandings of the role of bioethics. At a closer inspection it is not clear what kind of original question has started out the debate on bioethics. How does an ordinary problem or conflict become a bioethical problem? Since bioethics has been an interdisciplinary enterprise from its beginning, the different roles are defined from diverse professional perspectives. In order to see one's interests represented in the bioethical discourse, however, a certain language needs to be learnt. The ones who have shaped the language the most have gained the power of defining what counts as being a bioethical issue. They can be the winners in the game since they play the key role in setting the agenda around issues that deserve concern and public attention, and thus serve as a driving force to make the necessity for financial support convincible and political intervention unavoidable. The questions of justice and autonomy rather than responsibility and care, especially for the most vulnerable and dependent people have been put forward. Social circumstances and religious questions are mostly rendered invisible.

The Move of Bioethics into the Practical Arena: "Strangers at the Bedside"

Bioethicists are called upon to serve as expert consultants in numerous medical, legal, political, educational, and industrial arenas as well as the hospital arena. In addition to an analytical rationalistic style, and a technical procedure in the grasping process of ethical problem definition and going into a decision-making case, as pointed out before, applied pragmatism is also influential. Because professional practitioners and policy makers feel swamped, they call upon so-called 'bioethics experts', intellectuals and academics who help to resolve concrete problems in a reasonably clear way (Fox 1990: 209).

"This advisory role to decision makers has reinforced the cognitive predisposition of bioethics to distill the complexity and uncertainty, the dilemmas and the tragedy out of the situations they analyze. The fact that bioethicists are being asked to help professional practitioners and policymakers arrive at reasonably specific and clear ways of resolving the concrete medical-moral problems they face has given a new, expedient justification for the forms of intellectual and moral reductionism in which it engages" (Fox, Swazey 1984: 358).

The move from bioethics as an academic discipline into the hospital setting is described as a move from the "periphery to the center" (Chambers 2000: 22). Most scholars use the metaphor of inside – outside to describe the shift in bioethicists' work (Chambers 2000: 23). David Rothman for instance, identifies bioethicists as "strangers at the bedside" (Rothman 2003). He describes the movement as a history of how law and bioethics transformed clinical medical decision-making.[9]

DeVries and Conrad think that bioethics has been successful in altering the behaviour of physicians, medical researchers, administrators, and policy-makers, and that bioethicists would worry publicly about whether they are "watchdogs" or "lapdogs" (DeVries, Conrad 1998: 245). They doubt a forceful and troublesome presence of bioethics in medicine as well as a rather idealized view which claims that bioethicists represent the patient, protecting his or her autonomy against the power of the medical system. The authors see at least two organizational obstacles to a more powerful bioethics. First, greater authority might bring with it a moral 'deskilling' of physicians and other professionals in the decisions about care and responsibility for moral decisions could be transferred to bioethicists. The fear of *moral deskilling* has lead the Mayo Clinic to refuse bringing medical ethicists on staff. They regard every interaction between patient and caregiver as an ethical exchange. Therefore they insist all caregivers must be ethically skilled (DeVries, Conrad 1998: 246).[10] The second barrier that reduces the power of bioethicists is: "Ethicists reflect and physicians act. When the world of contemplation and ambiguity meets the world of action, the outcome is fixed. Ethicists lose. They are relegated to the sidelines" (DeVries, Conrad 1998: 246).

According to DeVries and Conrad, the presence of bioethicists in medical institutions might lead to an affinity between bioethicists and other professionals there (DeVries, Conrad 1998: 246). They remark: "The role of a bioethicist is in fact much like that of a public defender in the American legal system. The formal role of each is to represent the interests of a client in a large and confusing bureaucracy, many of whom are working against the interest of their clients" (DeVries, Conrad 1998: 246). DeVries and Conrad conclude: "Given this organizational situation, bioethicists will be inclined

---

9 I share Silja Samerski's (2002) remark that David Rothmann's historical work is the most critical in-depth study on the transformation process from experts to patients who decide, in the second half of the 20th century.

10 Instead of a staff of medical ethicists, they have created a medical humanities department that is responsible for organizing dramatic readings, plays, and film representations intended to make the Mayo staff ethically sensitive.

to represent the interests of medical professionals and medical institutions over those who are merely passing through – patients and families" (DeVries, Conrad 1998: 246).

As has already been pointed out before (see 1.3), the shape of bioethics and its definition of problems often implies an exclusion of political, social and communal matters of concern. Fox gives an apparent example, drawn from the context of the Neonatal Intensive Care Unit (NICU). She explains that bioethical attention was put on the

"[…] justifiability of non-treatment decisions, but relatively little attention has been paid to the fact that a disproportionately high number of extremely premature infants of very low birth weight, with severe congenital abnormalities, cared for in NICUs are babies born to poor, disadvantaged mothers, many of whom are single teenagers, and also nonwhite" (Fox 1990: 208).

And Fox states: "[…] these kinds of social problems are 'de-listed' as ethical problems in a manner that removes them from the sphere of moral scrutiny and concern" (Fox 1990: 208).

Chambliss, Fox, DeVries and Conrad observed that bioethicists ignore certain obvious questions about the structure of health care and the lack of sensitivity prevents American bioethicists from seeing the way they protect the status quo. In this context, Chambliss refers to Hospital Ethics Committees:

"Talk of 'ethical dilemmas' diverts attention from the structural condition that have produced the problem in the first place. This is naturally in the interest of the status quo and is relatively unthreatening to powerful interests within the hospital. This is why so many hospitals can readily accept an 'ethics committee' and its debates about ethical issues. Initially, some powerful hospital staff may feel threatened, but the threat is contained by framing issues as 'difficult dilemmas' rather than seeing them as symptoms of the structural flaws of the health care system" (Chambliss 1996: 92–93).

For Chambliss it is clear that bioethicists as well as ethics committees serve the interest of medical organizations (Chambliss 1996: 93).

Raymond DeVries and Peter Conrad share the critique given by Paul Wolpe that the individualistic stance of American bioethics leaves unchallenged the existing system of medicine (Wolpe 1998). The creation of an ethics for managed care could be regarded as one illustration of the structural blind spot. "The work of ethicists centers on discovering ways to determine what sorts of treatments the 'risk pool' can bear: When 300,000 people pool their resources for medical care, can they afford to pay for certain very expensive but experimental treatments?" (DeVries, Conrad 1998: 237). The authors ask, where the bioethical spotlight might be trained. With regard to hospitals, they identified a strong bioethical presence when entering: "The ethical stakes are higher there; it is a place where decisions with immediate and profound ethical consequences are made routinely" (DeVries, Conrad 1998: 235). But even here, in the practical arena of the hospital, DeVries and Conrad realized that not all spheres of potential ethical conflicts attract attention: For them, the ignorance of the inherent ethical questions in nursing practice exemplify the observance of inattention. The feminist journalist, Suzanne Gordon, who has been writing eloquently of the important role nurses play in health care, believes that in the midst of their routine care, nurses make "[...] profound ethical decisions" (Gordon 1997: 84). To illustrate her statement, she tells the story of a nurse who resisted the order of physicians to remove the catheter of a woman dying of cancer. The physicians were concerned about the danger of a urinary tract infection and removing the catheter would make the treatment of the infection easier. From the nurse's point of view, this handling was of no point and cruel, because it would cause severe pain and whether it would prolong the patient's life for some days nobody could tell (Gordon 1997: 84). DeVries and Conrad state: "[...] bioethicists do not see the important role played by nurses in ethical decision making. Somehow the ethical resonant work done by nurses is not labelled 'bioethical'. Nursing ethics is a minor planet in the galaxy of bioethics, offering its practitioners little respect and prestige" (DeVries, Conrad 1998: 235).[11]

Bioethical ways of framing a moral dilemma often put the bioethicist on the side of medicine. This tendency is illustrated by Judith Andre's story of a laboring woman who locked herself in a hospital bathroom in an effort to realize her desire for a non-medicated birth. After arranging for a drug-free birth with her obstetrician, she was shocked to be confronted with a nurse insisting on starting an intravenous line. Andre points out that the typical bioethical response to this dilemma is to define the problem as a "maternal-fetal conflict". The actions of the mother are seen as a threat to her child (and its 'autonomy'), not as an act of resistance to the medical system (Andre 2002).

---

11 Daniel Chambliss's literature review on the basic texts of bioethics has found out that nursing is mentioned very seldom. He draws the conclusion, that medical ethics is primarily focused on physicians and that nursing "[...] which will actually carry out many of the decisions (made by physicians), has no place in the discussion" (1996: 4–5).

In sum, the social science critique claims that the way bioethics has been shaped by Western philosophical rationalistic thought, social and cultural factors have been relegated to the status of irrelevancies. By focusing on individuals, the conceptual framework of bioethics plays down their inter-relationships, rationalizes and simplifies the emotional and the social and limits the range of facts and values considered germane to ethics. Bioethics is oriented to problem solving and decision making, and not engaged in understanding processes that might have created the problem. Questions that show an interest in the historical and cultural context of problems as well as political and social forces are hardly raised. Nevertheless, bioethicists' activities surround public spheres as well as private domains in which beliefs, values and norms are basic to society's cultural tradition, embedded in history.

2 Traces and Beginnings of Consultation by Committees

In analogy to the statement by Renee Fox that "Bioethics has never been just Bioethics", I will argue here that Institutional Ethics Committees – whether with regard to consultation, or with regard to research – have never been just Institutional Ethics Committees. There is no doubt that contemporary Hospital Ethics Committees evolved in the United States, but:

"Origins are difficult to trace with precision. How beginnings are located, what counts as an institutional antecedent to IECs, and what forerunners are ignored to us more about the intent of the analyst than it informs us about IECs. If the analyst tells the story in such a way that IECs are seen as an extension of earlier organizational forms, then one can expect a Whig history of medical ethics" (Bosk, Frader 1998: 96).

The idea of (formally) authorizing small groups of professionals and experts to make ethical decisions or give recommendations concerning medical treatment is not a new one. Where to start with the history of Clinical Ethics Committees and how to define this organized forum to discuss "ethical" issues in a hospital is not clear at all. Nevertheless, the concept of constituting a special committee to consider medical problems as well as medical intervention that are charged being "ethical" problems is not a new phenomenon.

Traces of Institutionalized Consultation Committees

As early as 1913 a Committee on Eugenics organized by the American Breeder's Association Committees delivered criteria for involuntary sterilization (Reilly 1991). As Jana Grekul, Harvey Krahn and Dave Odynak (2004) found out, for the sterilization of the "Feeble-minded" in Alberta, Canada from 1929 to 1972 an "Eugenics Board" was involved. Studying the Norwegian eugenics movement in the 1920s and 1930s (Broberg, Roll-Hansen 2005), the tendency to build up a forum of shared decision making can also be traced back. In Germany during World War II the Nazi medical committees decided on the subjects of sterilization and euthanasia.

Sterilization Committees as Eugenics Committees

Segregation as well as sterilization laws and programs were implemented in several states of the USA by the late 1800s. As Philip Reilly (1991) found out, over the next half decade, close to thirty states performed sterilization operations under their eugenic laws.

The history of involuntary sterilization can provide an illustration of the relationship between social processes and medical intervention. In the late nineteenth century a series of currents converged to give rise to the belief that the very character of American society was threatened by the increasing numbers of

"[...] degenerate persons whose biological traits predisposed them to lives of crime, idleness, poverty, dependency, alcoholism, insanity, idiocy, and disease generally. A faith that culture was shaped by biology rather than environment coloured the responses of many Americans who believed that the increase in degeneracy from both indigenous and foreign sources menaced the stability, tranquillity, and well-being of their nation. By the turn of the century, the pervasive tide of fear had already begun to shape public policies. The segregation of allegedly degenerate persons in institutions was common practice" (Grob 1991: ix).

Based on archival materials, the medical doctor and lawyer, Philip Reilly documented in his book the *Surgical Solution* the practice of involuntary sterilization programs that existed in the majority of the states. He found out that the courts approved them, and that they continued to function long after the eugenics had been discredited. This medical intervention by surgical techniques represented an effort to "uplift society by preventing the propagation of persons whose socially undesirable behaviour supposedly resulted from a deficient biological inheritance" (Grob 1991: x).

In 1906, the American Breeder's Association (ABA) had spawned forty-three committees, including one on eugenics that issued a report advocating surgical sterilization of persons identified as potential parents of defective children (Reilly 1991: 58). Due to the ABA's growing interest in the problem of racial degeneration, it established a special committee to "Study and to Report on the Best Practical Means of Cutting off the Defective Germ

Plasm in the American Population. The five-man committee was chaired by Bleeker Van Wagenen, the prominent New York attorney. Harry Laughlin, the only other nonphysician, was named as its secretary" (Reilly 1991: 59).

At the 1913 meeting of ABA, the committee report was delivered and enumerated "[…] classes (that) must generally be considered as socially unfit and their supply should if possible be eliminated from the human stock if we would maintain or raise the level of quality essential to the progress of the nation and our race" (Reilly 1991: 59).[12] Of the possible solutions, ranging from segregation to euthanasia, to the problem of "defective germ plasm" that the *committee* considered, it favored sterilization as the "least objectionable and most cost-effective method" (Reilly 1991: 60). Philip Reilly analyzed four decades of survey data and summary statistics on involuntary sterilization. In sum, his conclusions are that more than sixty thousand persons were sterilized under state laws between 1907 and 1963. The sterilization programs were most active during the 1930s, but in several states major sterilization programs were active in the 1940s and 1950s. From 1930 until the early 1960s sterilizations were performed on many more institutionalized women than men (Reilly 1991: 94). And: "Revulsion over Germany's racist politics did little to curtail American programs before or after World War II. Indeed, American advocates pointed to Germany to illustrate how an enlightened sterilization program might quickly reach its goals" (Reilly 1991: 95). During the 1940s there was a remarkable decline in the number of institutionalized persons that were sterilized each year in the United States. According to Reilly this was mainly caused by the shortage of civilian physicians during World War II. Despite an increase of eugenic sterilizations after the war, in most states they did not outnumber the prewar levels.

Jana Grekul, Harvey Krahn and Dave Odynak (2004) studied the sterilization of the " 'Feeble-minded': Eugenics in Alberta, Canada" from 1929 to 1972. With regard to a *collective decision-making process by an institutional organizational form*, they found out the following: When the *Sexual Sterilization Act* was passed in 1928 it allowed under certain conditions for the sterilization of inmates of mental health institutions. "A four-person Eugenics Board was created to determine if sterilization was appropriate for each case considered. Board members had to unanimously agree before sterilization was authorized. In addition, the patient had to give her / his consent,

---

12 Among these classes were people declared to be feeble minded, epileptics, constitutionally weak as well as persons born with marked criminal tendencies (Reilly 1991: 59).

unless they were mentally incapable. If so, the consent of a next of kin had to be obtained" (Grekul, Krahn, Odynak 2004: 363). The Eugenics Board began its work in 1929 and several years later their "success" was documented: "After reporting how many operations had been performed in only four years" there were authors who applauded the efficient manner in which the Sexual Sterilization Act was implemented and the Eugenics Board continued its operations until 1972 while the Alberta's *Sexual Sterilization Act* remained in force (Grekul, Krahn, Odynak 2004: 363 364). Sterilization was seen as the "only rational procedure" for dealing with mental defectives (Grekul, Krahn, Odynak 2004: 363). The *Sexual Sterilization Act* required that the Eugenics Board have four members, including the chairperson. Two members were supposed to be physicians. First a philosopher served as chair and later a physician. "Over 43 years, only 19 other individuals served as Board members. Most were professionals (medical doctors, psychiatrists, social workers)" (Grekul, Krahn, Odynak 2004: 363). Patients were "presented" to the Board by a representative of the institution in which they were cared for. Usually this representative was a medical doctor respectively a psychiatrist. The board members would interview the presented patients by relying on the presentation summary sheets prepared in advance. In case patients were unable to attend the meeting, the Board could visit them on the ward (at the bedside) to observe and ask questions. "Final decisions about sterilization were usually made at the same meeting, although sometimes decisions were deferred until additional information was available. On average the Board discussed 13 cases per meeting. This translates into, at best, about 13 minutes of Board discussion for each sterilization recommendation" (Grekul, Krahn, Odynak 2004: 363).

In 1972 the conservative government was to repeal the Act and dismantle the Eugenics Board. When a women who had been sterilized as a teenager successfully sued the Alberta government and won a settlement, only little more was heard about the activities of the Board (Grekul, Krahn, Odynak 2004: 364).

Looking at Norwegian eugenics movement in the 1920s and 1930s, the tendency to build up a forum of shared decision making can also be traced back: The Norwegian Consultative Eugenics Committee sent a proposal to the Ministry of Justice in 1931. Principles were described that the committee thought should form the basis of a law and not a concrete proposal for a law text (Broberg, Roll-Hansen 2005: 170). Although the committee was "little more that a paper organisation with a letterhead, [...] its public influence should not be underestimated. Its effect as a pressure group consisting of prominent citizens may have been considerable, and it did at least give [...] (the committees') activities some legitimacy" (Broberg, Roll-Hansen 2005: 170–171). The Consultative Eugenics Committee also formulated a draft for a sterilization law. In a statement written in 1933 for the medical faculty of the university at the request of the Ministry of Justice, Ragnar Vogt compared the proposal with that of his own commission and the newly introduced German law, *Gesetz zur Verhütung erbkranken Nachwuchses*. He emphasized that the proposal, like German law, was based on a principle of compulsory sterilization in contrary to the voluntary sterilization that his commission had proposed (Broberg, Roll-Hansen 2005: 172–173).

Catholic Medico-Moral Committees as Moral Protection Committees

The development of Clinical Ethics Committees in confessional organizations started in the 1920s when Catholic hospitals established bodies that were called Catholic Medico-Moral Committees (Levine 1984: 9). In 1949 the Catholic Hospital Organization (CHO) published the "Ethical and Religious Directives" for the first time (Jonsen 1998: 362–365). The text tried to convince Catholic hospitals to establish Multidisciplinary Ethics Committees. The main intention was to keep the norms of Catholic doctrine with regard to questions on e.g. contraception, abortion, and euthanasia under control (Steinkamp, Gordijn 2003: 96).

This showed that an organization reacted notably sensitively and explicitly to questions of its identity (given by alternative way of actions). Their interest was not to develop new patterns of argumentation with reference to new questions, but to protect a certain moral understanding. Is such a "moral bonding" still possible in today's committees?

Norbert Steinkamp and Bert Gordijn think that this could only happen in a very limited sense since today's expectations are different and do imply practical recommendations with regard to the organizational level. Moreover a greater autonomy of the committee that allows plurality of moral convictions would be expected (Steinkamp, Gordijn 2003: 95). Steinkamp and Gordijn found out that according to Jonsen (1998) the later versions of the *Ethical and Religious Directives* as well as the regulations of denominational committees have considered this (Steinkamp, Gordijn 2003: 95).

Steinkamp and Gordijn remark that the official clerical morale is regarded as an established and unquestioned body of concrete norms. Therefore their procedure of dealing with ethical questions in institutions is mainly deductive. Moral problems are analyzed in such a way that the "suitable piece" of the standing norms can be applied to the concrete situations in practice (Steinkamp, Gordijn 2003: 95).

According to a summary about empirical studies on Catholic Hospital Ethics Committees by Joan Kalchbrenner, Margaret Kelly and John Kelly (1983), these Catholic committees appear to have representatives and chairmen from a greater number of disciplines than do other ethics committees in US-hospitals overall. With regard to committee function, Catholic committees are found to be generally proactive and educational, rather than reactive, or problem-oriented (Kalchbrenner; Kelly, M.; Kelly, J. 1983: 49). Moreover: "Although ethics committees' major concern has been medical-moral issues, institutions are also focusing on social justice issues [...]" (Kalchbrenner, Kelly, M.; Kelly, J. 1983: 50)

Abortion Review Committees as Control Committees

In 1945 the Abortion Review Committees were founded by Alan Guttmacher (Moreno 1995: 97). Defenders of the committees argued that they would act in the patient's best interests, provide physicians with a medico-legal safeguard, and serve as a repository of data about interrupted pregnancies. Opponents of Abortion Review Committees argued that they "[...] were a smokescreen for physicians who wished to protect themselves from public criticism" (Moreno 1995: 95). Others charged that any particular committee could be constituted so that abortions were virtually banned or virtually unrestricted.

By the mid-1950s, according to Rickie Solinger, in many non-Catholic hospitals, physicians assembled themselves collectively into abortion boards or committees. "As a group", Solinger explains "obstetricians, cardiologists, psychiatrists, and others considered abortion recommendations and requests and issued definitive decisions on each case" (Solinger 1993: 248).

"These committees protected physicians, individually and as a profession, in a number of ways. Of paramount importance to many was the legal protection the boards provided. Four medical doctors, characterizing the therapeutic abortionist as a 'fetal executioner', stressed that group review of all cases was crucial because the 'legal burden' otherwise rested on the individual obstetrician" (Solinger, Rickie 1993: 249).

In 1973 the United States Court affirmed in a revolutionary decision (called Roe v. Wade decision) the constitutional right to abortion. The thrust of Roe v. Wade was to maximize privacy and parental autonomy in that a woman who wanted a fetus aborted had the right to do so. "In this way, Roe v. Wade expanded the domain of private decision making against both professional and state authority, and thus was most consistent, in the context of newborns and termination of treatment […]" (Rothman 2003: 204). According to Brendan Minogue (1996), only few judical decisions have caused more conflict and controversy in the United States (Minogue 1996: 198). "Did one begin by discounting the life of the fetus and then move, inexorably, to discounting the life of the newborn, and, eventually the elderly?" (Rothman 2003: 205). Betty Sarvis and Hyman Rodman wrote on behalf of the committees that they would clearly serve a purpose for hospitals in a situation where little consensus can be achieved and where the law leaves the decision in medical hands (Sarvis, Rodman 1974).

"In fact, however, considerable consensus seems to have been achieved within the committees themselves – even if not in society – or at least not deep differences in points of view among the members were reported. This could be attributed either to professional etiquette in not publicizing such differences, or to a deliberate selection of members among the committees in the proportion of rejected requests for abortions, ranging from 25 percent at one California hospital to 60 percent at another" (Moreno 1995: 96).

According to George Annas and Michael Grodin (1993), abortion committees were the first committees that might be termed ethics committees because they had been set up by statutes to review abortion decisions. This was the time when most states had statutes that forbade abortions. An exception was made if a hospital abortion committee had found the pregnant woman's life to be in danger. Committees were the most popular method for determining who would be able to have a therapeutic abortion (Levine 1984: 9).

It is explicit in the literature and documents that abortion committees had only doctors as members and made medical judgements about whether or not a patient's medical condition fit the state definition under which abortion could be performed legally. With regard to nurses' non-participation in abortion committees, it is important to note that the issue of conscientious objection has arisen in connection with abortion. Although abortions were legal there were nurses who objected to them on grounds of conscience (Jameton 1984: 286). Therefore, the International Labor Conference recommended that nursing personnel should be able to claim exemption from performing specific duties, without being penalized, where performances would conflict with their religious, moral, or ethical convictions (Jameton 1984: 286–287). Placing conscientious objection historically in the context of abortion leaves the question, why sterilization had not been an issue of conscientious objection for nurses.

Kidney Dialysis Committees as Selection Committees

In 1960, when Belding Scribner, a medical doctor at the University of Washington, Seattle, invented a medical device called a shunt, it revolutionized the treatment of chronic kidney disease, that is also known as end-stage renal failure. The newly developed plastic shunt could be more or less permanently implanted in the patient's vein. Since the tubes of the dialysis unit could enter the patient's veins over and over again through the shunt, dialysis could be performed repeatedly as long as the patient would need it. And the patient would need it as long as he lived.

The era of long-term dialysis began: the device made it possible to treat chronic renal disease by long-term haemodialysis. In other words, the shunt apparatus cured no disease, but made long-treatment possible on an artificial kidney machine. "It is the prototypical success story of modern medicine: Where there had been certain death, now there was continued life, although of reduced quality" (Winslade, Ross 1986: 23). Anyone could have benefited from this technological progress. Kidney failure is, for example, not a disease of the elderly. It is the product of many diseases, mostly a result of hypertension. The problem: There were by far more patients than the equipment could handle. Furthermore, the treatment was extremely expensive – more than most patients could pay (Ross 1986: 24). Katz and Proctor resume: Although between 1960 and 1972 both dialysis and renal transplantation had become applicable, more long-term and effective, extraordinary forms of therapy for end-stage chronic kidney disease, there were not enough machines, trained personnel, medical centers to treat all, or even most of the patients in this condition (Katz, Proctor 1969). "The new hopes generated by Scibners's shunt were muted, [...] when hospitals were faced with the problem of deciding which patients were to receive dialysis – and live – and which ones were to be rejected – and die" (Winslade, Ross 1986: 24). To deal with the increasing "allocation" problems, a special committee on chronic kidney disease, later called "Kidney Dialysis Selection Committee" was appointed by the federal government (Fox 1989: 131).

"These scarcity / selection /allocation problems, along with the choices that could now be made between in-center and home dialysis, live-related and cadaveric renal transplants, and various combinations of them, also contributed to the quality of life and quality of death questions with which the medical profession, patients with kidney disease, their families, the public, and the polity became progressively concerned" (Fox 1989: 133).

Renee Fox and Judith Swazey (1974) underline that it is worth noting that such committees faced enormous pressures trying to reach consensus, never articulated standards for decision-making, and eventually disbanded, an outcome perhaps helped along by considerable adverse publicity. An important feature of these groups was the sharp focus on case-by-case decisions. The committees after all functioned as clinical consultants. Neither the social rules that structured the consultation nor the philosophical and social value assumptions that shaped the decisions were explicit.

In Seattle, the Swedish hospital in which Scribner was working, a forum that was called "Treatment Committee" was formed. The committee reviewed cases of patients who were medically qualified for dialysis and selected the ones with the best prognosis. "Biomedical criteria were used, but given the 'state of the art' and medical 'problems of uncertainty', only the roughest kind of consensus existed about indications and contradictions in this regard" (Fox 1989: 133). Some patients were rejected because they did not meet the criteria given by physicians: They were either too young (because dialysis would severely retard their growth and development), too old (to benefit), or they had other major diseases (like severe diabetes, cardiovascular disease, and carcinoma) that made success with dialysis less likely (Ross 1986: 6).

In 1967, the survey by Katz and Proctor reported that only half of the dialysis centers in the United States had explicit medical criteria for selecting or rejecting a patient (Katz, Proctor 1969). Renee Fox remarks: "The problem of deciding which treatment a kidney patient should receive preoccupied the medical profession as much as the questions of who should be treated, who not, and who should make that decision" (Fox 1989: 134). Jonathan Moreno's research on these committees revealed that they found the middle-aged male bank officer with a wife and three children to be a superior candidate, in comparison to the older person who is unemployed, a former alcoholic and has no dependents (Moreno 1995: 96). The so called "psychological and social suitability criteria" tended to blur over into social background, social status and "social worth" considerations (Fox 1989: 133).

Winslade and Ross report about the "Treatment Committee of St. Anne's Community Hospital" without giving the location.

"The committee included six members, two doctors (one a psychiatrist), one hospital administrator, one nurse, and a clergyman and a lawyer from the community. Except for the committee themselves, only the hospital director knew who was on the committee. The decision to form the committee had been handled quietly and there had been no reason to identify the prospective members publicly. Then, after the first meeting, they had requested that their identities be kept secret because they feared that prospective patients would seek them out to argue for their lives. It had seemed a sensible request to the director for other reasons as well: if the hospital were going to ask the members to decide who was to live and who to die, it did not need to burden them additionally by making them publicly accountable for their choices" (Winslade, Ross 1986: 27).

Moreover, the committee members decided never to see the patients nor their physicians. First, in order not to be identified, and second, so that their decisions would not be inappropriately or emotionally biased (Winslade, Ross 1986: 27).

The selection processes were repeated in hospitals throughout the United States during the years between 1962 and 1972. According to Fox, Winslade and Ross, physicians, nurses, social workers, psychologists, psychiatrists, and, in certain centers, clergymen, lawyers and lay people participated in the selection committees that were made up. In the literature nothing is said about the possibly unique roles of the different professions. Even though physicians expressed the usual reservations about lay intrusions in the doctor-patient relationship, by that time it had been widely appreciated that the decisions involved went beyond individual professional-client relationships (Moreno 1995: 96). As the Katz and Proctor study showed, however, the predominant role in voting on patient selection was acted out by physicians, the primary gatekeepers (Katz, Proctor 1969).

There has not been any study on the different perspectives in the multidisciplinary committees and their way of working and making decisions. Moreno suggests considering that the committee members were operating on two levels of consensus.

"The first was the level of the values that they brought with them into the room, values that in this case seemed to validate certain operating principles, albeit largely tacit and unarticulated principles. The second was the level of values that they manifested when they made specific decisions. When there were disagreements about these particular cases, they were forced to go back to their largely unexpressed background theory and see if they could find a reason for the disagreement that might also provide a shared basis for resolving it" (Moreno 1995: 97).

In 1962, *Life* magazine published an article by Shane Alexander *"They Decide Who Lives, Who Dies"* which described, though anonymously, the operation of the selection committee at the Swedish Hospital in Seattle. The story provoked widespread comment, and disapproval was expressed about committees "playing God" (Winslade, Ross 1986: 32–33; Dzur 2002: 181). It had proved to be obvious that individuals were being selected for treatment (and thus for life) on the basis of criteria related to social worth and consequently, the Seattle program was charged of ethical insensitivity. But: "The number of people directly affected by the availability of dialysis was [...] too small to create any kind of political force, especially since they were not concentrated in any single geographical area" (Winslade, Ross 1986: 33).

By 1972, the federal government could no longer ignore the issue. The US Public Health Service established a research program and funded kidney dialysis demonstration programs. Public Health was to provide an initial three-year funding; then the centers had to find other fundings. The federal government's slow response had made the problem an intensely personal one for those who needed treatment.

Judith Ross thinks of the possibility that some hospitals maintained or created treatment committees afterwards, using them to discuss ethical considerations in clinical care, but, "[...] if so, the committees did not leave any published records of their activities" (Ross 1986: 3*)*.

From Professional Ethical Standards to Governmental Intervention

The Military Tribunal in Nuremberg which tried the Nazi physicians formulated a code of ethics that has shaped medical research of post-World War II. One major contribution of the code was to make the voluntary consent of the human subject absolutely fundamental.[13] The duty and responsibility for ascertaining the quality of the consent rests upon each individual who is in any way involved in the experiment. This personal responsibility may not be delegated to somebody else. The code declares that the experiment should be such as to yield fruitful results for the good of society and

---

13 There are other codes, including a 1931 German Interior Ministry document, expressing the necessity to respect individual human subjects (Annas, Grodin 1993).

not be procurable by other methods or means of study and not trivial or unnecessary in nature.

During the course of the experiment, the human subject on the one hand, should be at liberty to end his participation if he reaches the physical or mental state where continuation seems to the person impossible. The scientist on the other hand, must be prepared to terminate the experiment at any stage if he realizes that a continuation is likely to result in injury, disability, or even death for the experiment's subject.[14]

In 1953, the National Institutes of Health developed procedures to regulate research conducted at its clinical center (Faden, Beauchamp 1986) and since the early 1960s several institutions had created *Institutional Review Boards* (IRBs) on their own initiative (Moreno 1995:97). Medical research in hospitals as well as other health care institutions created more and more open questions that were identified as ethical problems. When patients were used as subjects in these experiments, problems could include what comprised informed consent and what sorts of experiments ought not to be conducted even if subjects gave informed consent. Betty Sichel explains:

"For example, if one group of patients were to be given a medication that might alleviate symptoms of life-threatening illness and another sample with the same illness were given a placebo, should the experiment be permitted even if all patients give informed consent? The federal government was not concerned with the answer to the question, but with the method for making the decision" (1992:115).

It was commonly believed in the 1950s and 1960s that medical experiments in the United States were immune to abuse due to the high ethical standards of the profession (Jameton 1984: 108). However, in 1966 Henri Beecher, a Harvard medical professor, documented a number of questionable ethical studies (1966: 1354–1360). Among the most well known abuses that came to public attention thereafter was the *cancer immunology experimentation* at the Jewish Chronic Disease Hospital in New York. Physicians injected cancer cells into hospitalized elderly patients. They were not informed about it because the physicians thought if they were, they would not consent to the study. The physician wanted to study the immune response and were sure

---

14 The promulgation of other codes of ethics, such as the World Medical Association Helsinki Declaration (1964), the American Medical Association Ethical Guidelines for Clinical Investigation (1966), the American Nurses Association Human Rights Guidelines for Nurses in Clinical and Other Research (1975), have focused attention not only on the ethical dilemmas inherent in research activities but also on the limitation of codes (Davis et al. 1997: 109).

that the patients would not get cancer (Langer 1966: 663–66). What also came to public attention was the *hepatitis experiment on mentally retarded children* institutionalized at Willowbrook: Mentally retarded children were injected with hepatitis in order to study the disease. Often because parents could get earlier admission to the hospital, they consented (Gorovitz et al. 1976: 123–142). Moreover, there is the *Tuskegee syphilis research on African Americans* in the South to mention. The study began in the 1930s when rural black men were chosen as subjects in a longitudinal study of syphilis. Although a cure for syphilis was later found, it was decided not to treat the black men in order to complete the study (Reiser, Dyck, Curran 1977: 316–321). Not to forget the *"experimental pregnancy"* with Mexican-American women: The Mexican women were given placebo birth control pills to study the psychological side effects of oral contraceptives. Many became pregnant because they were not told of the placebo (Veatch 1971: 2–3).

When the scandals came to light, in 1971, the Department of Health, Education and Welfare (HEW)[15] appointed the first consecutive National Commission to report on bioethical questions in medicine and research. In July 1974, the National Research Act passed by US-Congress under the leadership of Walter Mondale[16] and Edward Kennedy the *National Commission for the Protection of Human Subjects of Biomedical and Behavioral Research* (hereafter the National Commission). It became temporary, rather than permanent, and advisory to the secretary of HEW, without any enforcement powers of its own (Rothman 2003: 189). This group, consisting of three physicians, three lawyers, two biomedical researchers, two ethicists, one member of the public, was charged with an investigation of medical ethics and to identify the basic ethical principles which should underlie the conduct of biomedical and behavioural research (Davis et al. 1997: 111; Fox 1990: 204). It then had to develop guidelines for ethical conduct and experimentation which were formulated in a policy for the protection of

---

15 The HEW is now the Department of Health and Human Services (DHHS).
16 In 1968, three months after Christiaan Barndard's surgical feat, Walter Mondale, then senator from Minnesota, introduced a bill to establish a Commission on Health Science and Society for the assessment and report on the ethical, legal, social, and political implications of biomedical advances (Rothman 2003: 168). He explained: "The scientific breakthrough of the last few months were current highlights in a dazzling half century of truly unprecedented advance in the medical and biological sciences […] These advances and others yet to come raised grave and fundamental ethical and legal questions for our society – who shall live and who shall die; how long shall life be preserved and how shall it be altered; who shall make decisions; how shall society be prepared" (quoted after Rothman 2003: 169).

human subjects that should be followed in such research to assure that it is conducted in accordance with such principles (Davis et al. 1997: 111; Fox 1990: 204, Rothman 2003: 168). Mondale had urged the establishment of a National Commission to serve as a forum in which not only doctors and biomedical researchers but, lay representatives would explore these issues together (Rothman 2003: 169). Fred Harris, Oklahoma senator who distrusted experts, shared Mondale's concerns. He declared that the bioethical matters should be talked in public by people from various backgrounds with various viewpoints: Theological as well as medical, legal as well as sociological and psychological (Rothman 2003: 169). Although the commission was not permanent and was charged to investigate not all of medicine but only human experimentation, it had a vital and continuing presence: Within the next three years, the Commission published a series of reports on several aspects of experimentation with "[...] special categories of human subjects from whom it is problematic to obtain informed consent: Human fetuses and pregnant women, children, prisoners, mentally ill or retarded persons who are institutionalized, and individuals who are possible candidates for psychosurgery" (Fox 1990: 204). The recommendations in the reports were the bases for the regulations governing "human experimentation", finally adopted by the Department of Health and Human Services.

By mid-1970s, federal rules were in place requiring the systematic review of government-sponsored research involving human subjects. The establishment of Institutional Review Boards was mandated in order to evaluate the acceptability of medical research with patients of health care institutions. These mandatory Institutional Committees in hospitals, medical centers, and other such facilities around the USA have been in charge of initial review of all research proposals and periodic review in order to ascertain that each researcher has outlined the risks and benefits and the subjects have given their informed consent to participate in the study. "Essentially, the IRB must determine that the rights and welfare of the subjects are protected, that the risks to an individual are outweighed by the potential benefit to him or her and society, and that informed consent will be obtained by adequate and appropriate methods" (Davis et al. 1997: 110).[17] With this mandating, health care workers realized that there was considerable precedent for federal government intervention (Fox 1990). In 1979, five years af-

---

17 These governmental review standards, although worded in general terms, do detail the basic elements of informed consent, thereby drawing importance to its importance (Davis et al. 1997: 110).

ter its founding, the National Commission issued an influential document, known as the *Belmont Report* (Moreno 1995: 76).

The Belmont Report defined three principles: respect for persons, beneficience, and justice. These principles aimed at providing an analytical framework which should guide the resolution of ethical problems arising from research on human subjects. Nevertheless the climax of rationalistic, principled medical ethics really began with the first publication of Beauchamp and Childress's *Principles of Biomedical Ethics* (1983). Major territorial claims for the basic principles were mapped out during the late 1970s and dominated the discussion of medical ethics during the 1980s. "The problem of relying overly much on principles in medical ethics is that agreement on principles may not lead to agreement on conclusions, and agreement on conclusion may not imply an agreement on principles" (Thomasma 1994: 88). When a protest developed on the essential tidiness of an ethics of principles, it centered largely on an overreliance on the principle of autonomy. This led to an analysis of the strengths and weaknesses of an autonomy-based medical ethics. Both physicians, Edmund Pellegrino and David Thomasma (1988) have argued that it would leave out the essential person, the physician.

While setting forth the requirements for Institutional Review Boards, the Department of Health, Education and Welfare stated that diverse membership was important and should enhance the IRBs credibility. Moreover it would ensure sensitivity to the concerns of both investigators and human research subjects. No IRB could be entirely all male or all female, and a variety of racial and cultural groups had to be represented. In addition, the rules demanded that there must be at least a "non-scientific" member, as well as individuals representing several disciplines (Department of Health and Human Services 1981: 8375). That the spirit of these regulations has not yet been realized is shown in the studies by Bell, Whiton and Connelly (1998) as well as the study by Raymond DeVries and Carl Forsberg (2002). The studies show that the Review Boards have been dominated by (white) physicians and scientists, and only a comparable few number of nurses, other health care practitioners, lawyers, philosophers have been included (Gray 1975: 318–328).

The American Nurses' Association (ANA) code lists general guidelines outlining obligations of nurses' participation in research: First, to ascertain that the study design has been approved by an appropriate body. Second, to obtain information about the intent and nature of the research. Third, to determine whether the research is consistent with professional goals (ANA

1976).[18] Andrew Jameton remarks that nurses have been frequently aware of the moral ambiguities in research and have participated reluctantly in procedures they felt would not help the patient (1984: 110). Even though this calls for research on the composition, competence and work of ethics committees, there have only been a few studies generated (DeVries, Forsberg 2002: 252).

The sociological study by Raymond DeVries and Carl Forsberg (2002) looks at demographic and professional characteristics of members of IRBs. The results of the stratified random sample were: The mean size of the IRBs was 13 members with a relatively even distribution of gender across percentages, although 69 percent have less than half female members. 70 percent of the committees have at least 80 percent of white membership. Physicians account for 34 percent of all members, followed by 24 percent behavioural scientists, as well as 10 percent medical and biological scientists. Only 8 percent were nurses. DeVries and Forsberg remark that despite much criticism and several calls for reform, only little has changed since the mid-1990s. The membership of local committees still over-represents whites, medical researchers, and those affiliated with the sponsoring institution (2002: 255). The studies show that not all voices are adequately represented in IRB deliberation and that "the over-representation of certain voices may empower the interests and perspectives of researchers and research institutions relative to those of research subjects" (DeVries, Forsberg 2002: 256).

From the movement toward IRBs, in general, Moreno sees an appreciation at the federal level "[…] that decisions concerning human beings in research are not only purely scientific matters, but also they involve the consideration of moral values" (Moreno 1995: 97). The establishment of IRBs is distinctive in that it led to statutory requirements for an ethics committee review of processes which would formerly have been regarded strictly as matters of professional competence. Moreno stresses it as a significant fact that specific standards of judgement are imposed on all such bodies in the form of the three ethical principles (Moreno 1995: 98).

---

18 Andrew Jameton has summed up a number of precautions that nurses should keep in mind when they either conduct research or cooperate in research (1984: 110).

3 The Development of Contemporary Hospital Ethics Committees

In 1976, the New Jersey Supreme Court's decision in the case of Karen Ann Quinlan is seen as crucial for certifying the legal right of formerly competent patients to refuse treatment. This decision also reintroduced the topic of Hospital Ethics Committees.

The Story of Karen Quinlan

"The culmination of the decade-long process of bringing strangers to the bedside came in the case of Karen Quinlan. Its impact on opinion and policy outweighed even that of the scandals in human experimentation. [...] After Quinlan there was no disputing the fact that medical decision making was in the public domain and that a profession that had once ruled was now being ruled" (Rothman 2003: 222).

In April 1975 Karen Quinlan, at the age of twenty-two, was brought into the New Jersey hospital emergency room (Rothman 2003: 222). Though she was diagnosed irreversibly brain damaged and stated to be in a so called "persistent vegetative state", Karen Quinlan was not "brain-dead" and the etiology of her coma was never fully explained (Sichel 1992: 114).

After several months of hope, her parents recognized that she would not recover and they asked her physicians to remove her from the respirator which had been assisting her breathing. Her mother, Julia and her father, Joseph Quinlan, practicing Catholics, were looking for church guidance and had been told that taking Karen off the machine, even if she would then die was morally a correct action since this would return Karen to her "natural state" whereas respiratory care was seen as "extraordinary" (Rothman 2003: 222). According to the parent's account of events, St. Clair's hospital staff initially responded to their request to discontinue the treatment. The hospital made them sign a paper which declared that the responsible physician,

Dr. Morse, was authorized and directed to discontinue all extraordinary measures, including the use of a respirator for their daughter. The document noted that the physicians had explained all the consequences of the removal and were therefore released "from any and all liability". The parents were relieved, but the next day, Dr Morse called them to tell that he had a "moral problem" with the agreement, and that he intended to consult a colleague. When he called the day after, he informed them that he would not remove Karen from the respirator (Rothman 2003: 222–223). Rothman remarks:

"The staff would not even consider removing Karen from the respirator unless a court formally appointed them Karen's legal guardians. [...] Dr. Morse, and the other physicians who testified on his behalf, scrupulously differentiated between withholding treatment in the hopeless case, which was allowable, and withdrawing treatment from the hopeless case, which ostensibly was not" (Rothman 2003: 223–227).

The Quinlans went before the Superior Court of New Jersey to ask that the father (Joseph) be appointed Karen's guardian for the expressed purpose to request their child's removal from the respirator. When the Quinlans had begun to consider bringing the case to court, the lawyer warned them not only of the extensive publicity that was likely to follow, but also of the fact that the medical profession is a powerful one (Rothman: 2003: 224).

In November 1975, the lower court rejected the petition. The hospital reserved judgement, because due to any criteria, including the Harvard brain-death standards, Karen was alive; and disconnecting her from the respirator might well violate the ethical principle to "do no harm" as well as "[...] open the doctors and the hospital to criminal prosecution for homicide" (Rothman 2003: 223). The reason, concluded the court, had to do with physicians' fears of malpractice suits (Rothman 2003: 227). Betty Sichel remarks:

"The court justified its decision not to authorize removal of the respirator, noting that the rapid advancement of medical knowledge made it impossible to foresee what future knowledge would mean for the patient's health, recognizing the absence of medical tradition to warrant the act, and referring to legal precedent" (Sichel 1992: 114).

Then, the parents went before the State's Supreme Court which accepted the case. The justices wrestled with the problem of whether or not Quinlan's respirator could be disconnected. The court finally accepted the lawyer's (Paul Armstrong) argument, that a "[...] constitutionally protected right to privacy overlay the doctor-patient relationship" (Rothman 2003: 225).

As a consequence, the truly difficult issue turned to the question whether the court could dare to tell physicians how to treat, or not to treat, their patients. The relevance of this question is shown in the way, how the court transformed the idea of a *Multidisciplinary Committee* into a *Prognosis Committee* composed of physicians.

Multidisciplinary Advisory Committees as Physicians' Prognosis Committees

At the time when Karen Quinlan was raising wide attention, New Jersey's justices were impressed by a 1975 Baylor Law Review article written by Karen Teel, a pediatrician. The inspiration for the proposal of a local committee in the case of Karen Quinlan is taken from her.

"I see medical caretakers, the physicians, the nurses, and others whose whole orientation is assuming the sanctity of life and whose whole efforts are directed at preserving that life with every ounce of potential that can be realized, who then are faced with the reality of a no-win situation [...] I suggest that it would be more appropriate to provide a regular forum for more input and dialogue in individual situations and to allow the responsibility of these judgements to be shared [...] an Ethics Committee composed of physicians, social workers, attorneys, and theologians, [...] which serves to review the individual circumstances of ethical dilemma [...] (and) safeguards for patients and their medical caretakers. [...] Generally, the authority of these committees is primarily restricted to the hospital setting and their official status is more that of an advisory body than of an enforcing body" (Teel 1975: 9).[19]

Teel contended that physicians are charged with the responsibility of making ethical judgements for which they are sometimes "ill-equipped" on intellectual grounds and "knowingly or not, assumed civil and criminal liability" (Teel 1975: 8). The proposed multidisciplinary committee would not only bring a new and valuable dialogue to medical decision making process but from a legal point of view, share and divide responsibility (Teel 1975: 8).

Although Teel saw such a committee as being "advisory" rather than "enforcing", the New Jersey court had given it a greater role. In their land-

---

19 There have been Clinical Ethics Committees before official establishment as Teel points out.

mark decision they ruled that if Quinlan's attending physician determined that there was no "reasonable chance" that she would ever return to a "cognitive, sapient state", and if a Hospital Ethics Committee agreed with that prognosis, then the life supporting apparatus could be withdrawn at her guardian's or family's request on the basis of an individual's right of privacy. With this sort of mechanism, the physician would be immune from civil or criminal liability (Cranford, Doudera 1984: 14). Recognizing that the constitutional right of privacy applied to the refusal of medical treatment, the court held the opinion that Karen Quinlan's right to privacy should not be surrendered because she was "incompetent" (Murphy 1989: 552).

The judge at the Supreme Court had understood something very different than Karen Teel meant. Although the court had taken up her suggestion and called for a Hospital Ethics Committee, as a way to serve and protect hospitals by reviewing the individual circumstances of the dilemma, to assist families and helping physicians in reaching appropriate decisions, it did not show any interest in its multidisciplinary character: "The court's concept of an ethics committee was to consist wholly of physicians [...]" (Moreno 1995: 98). Their assumption where to settle an "ethical dilemma" was put on the basis of medical descriptions and definitions and charging it to decide no other issues of a case, but the narrower technical questions of whether the patient was in a chronic "vegetative state" or whether any "reasonable" chance of recovery existed (Rothman 2003: 228). As noted by Norman Fost and Ronald Cranford the expression Hospital Ethics Committee in this case was a misnomer since what they really intended was a *neurological diagnosis* given by medical experts (Fost, Cranford 1985: 2688). Betty Sichel remarks: "Expert medical knowledge alone could determine what decision should be made [...]" (1992: 114). Thus, the court was transforming Teel's multidisciplinary advisory committee into a *Physicians' Prognosis Committee*.

Afterwards the talk about ethics committees subsided. In many hospitals, however, some doctors, nurses, hospital administrators, and social workers started to meet regularly in small groups to discuss clinical problems they were facing, attended conferences on ethical problems in health care and addressed the problems with their colleagues. They called themselves *Bioethics Study Groups* and worked mostly unknown (Purtillo 2005, see Appendix 1.1).

The philosopher and clinical ethicist, Ruth Purtilo who declares herself to be "a piece of the history of Ethics Committees in the United States" tells: "After some time, they took on a more formal role in the hospital and began to provide education programs within the institution and worked on guidelines that would help to make decision making less traumatic" (Purtilo 2005, see Appendix 1.1). She is convinced that "[...] it is Boston where it all began with the ethics committee movement" (Purtilo 2005, see Appendix 1.1). Therefore, it deserves a closer look at what happened in Boston at the Massachusetts General Hospital (MGH).

Types of Hospital Ethics Committees: From Ad hoc Committee to Optimum Care Committee at Boston Massachusetts General Hospital

"With public scrutiny heightened, a few hospitals took steps to bring greater formality to the decision-making process. The Quinlan decision became the occasion for setting up committees to advise and review termination decisions and to formulate guidelines for individual physicians. Thus, the Massachusetts General Hospital administrators appointed an ad hoc committee to study 'how best to manage the hopelessly ill patient [...]'" (Rothman 2003: 229).

In the beginning of the 1970s the Massachusetts General Hospital administrators appointed a psychiatrist, two physicians, a nursing administrator, a lay person and a "legal counsel" to an ad hoc committee. Its task was to study how "best to manage the hopelessly ill patient" (Rothman 2003: 229; Purtilo 2005, see Appendix 1.1). The committee recommended a classification system, especially for patients with brain death or when there was no reasonable possibility that the patient would return to a cognitive and sapient life. This four-point patient-classification system, then established by MGH, ranged from A: Meaning "maximal therapeutic effort without reservation" to D: Meaning "all therapy can be discontinued" (Rothman 2003: 229). However, Troyen Brennan found out by reviewing medical records, that the original prognosis classification scheme was not strictly followed (Brennan 1988: 803). Although Brennan does not give an explanation, one could assume that the guidelines probably did not meet what the situation of the individual patient demanded. The Beth Israel Hospital, also in Boston, referred to Quinlan and drew up guidelines for ordering a DNR (Do Not Resuscitate) code for a patient.

"When a physician believed a patient to be 'irreversibly and irreparably ill', with death 'imminent' (that is, likely to occur within two weeks), the physician could elect to discuss with an ad hoc committee, composed exclusively of doctors, whether death was so certain that resuscitation would serve no purpose. If the committee members unanimously agreed, and the competent patient made it his or her 'informed choice', then a DNR order would be entered in the patient's chart; should the patient be incompetent, the physician was to obtain the approval of the family and then enter the order" (Rothman 2003: 230).

These measures were implemented with great caution and not readily adopted in other settings. Most hospitals did not adopt guidelines and resisted establishing committees.

In 1974, Boston Massachusetts Hospital turned its adhoc-committee into an Institutional Ethics Committee, called the *Optimum Care Committee* (OCC). Its task was to deal with end of life care and intervention "in situations where difficulties arise in deciding the appropriateness of continuing intensive therapy for critically ill patients" (Rothman 2003: 230). The members were a surgeon, an internist who was also a lawyer, and the chairperson, a psychiatrist with a divinity degree. Purtilo remarks: "There was also a nurse, but it was physician dominated" (Purtilo 2005, see Appendix 1.1). "The OCC nurse gathers information on patient status, the attitudes of family members, and the opinions of the nursing staff about the limitation or withdrawal of care" (Brennan 1988: 803). The committee did only meet at the request of the attending physician who had to record the prognosis for the patient. Then, the committee role was advisory: Its members consulted with one another, sometimes as a group and sometimes by telephone, and discussed the case. "They are guided mainly by a principle of beneficience, asking what would be the best thing to do for the patient" (Brennan 1988: 803). The recommendation that was worked out, went back to the physician, who was free to accept or reject its advice.

From 1974 through 1986, the committee's seventy-three consultations represented a broad experience with the problems that arose when care for terminally ill patients was limited. Brennan, committee participant evaluated the collected data in an article, called *Ethics Committees and Decisions to Limit Care. The Experience at the Massachusetts General Hospital* (1988). It appeared that more families had been requesting that care be withdrawn when there was no hope of recovery. Many physicians hesitated to defer to the family's wish that mechanical ventilatory support or hydration to be stopped. In many cases there was no family, or the family members were far away and would not make a decision on behalf of their relative. In other situations, the family was divided, and some families wanted no limitations on care despite the fact that the patient was clearly not going to recover (Brennan 1988: 806). However, the court deferred judgement on issue of DNR status when the family and the physician disagreed (Brennan 1988: 807). Brennan remarks: "[...] the role of ethics committees in making these decisions is not clear. It is not easy to say whether an ethics committee should recommend that physicians overrule family wishes on the assumption that a rational person would opt for DNR status if terminally ill and incompetent" (Brennan 1988: 807). Finally, Brennan concludes based on the ten-year committee experience:

"The experience of the OCC at the Massachusetts General Hospital is valuable because it provides a model for an ethics committee's role in limited care cases and highlights the questions that arise in such cases. No one person can provide answers to these questions. Rather, they must be addressed by ethicists, lawyers, judges, physician, and thoughtful members of our society [...]" (Brennan 1988: 807).

In 1977, a so-called "bioethics committee" was formed at the Montefiore Medical Center in New York that served primarily as an educational, policy-making, as well as guideline-writing consultative committee "responsible directly to the president of the medical center" (Rosner 1985: 2694).

Robert Veatch (1977) assessed the role of the committees and came to differentiate between four different types: (1) committees to review ethical and other values in individual patient care decisions, (2) committees to make larger ethical and policy decisions, (3) counselling committees, and (4) prognosis committees. He remarks that it would still be unclear which types will gain support and how they will evolve. The issues they pose would be significant ones, and their resolution would merit further study (Veatch 1977).

The President's Commission and its
Support of Hospital Ethics Committees

When the mandate of the National Commission for the Protection of Human Subjects was about to expire in 1978, it was transformed into the *President's Commission for the Study of Ethical Problems in Medicine and Medical and Bio-behavioural Research* (hereafter the President's Commission). The United States Congress charged the Commission to provide a temporary, national body that would consider the problematic situations that had arisen in medicine primarily, but not exclusively, as a result of advances in medical technology (Ross 1986: 18–19; Rothman 2003: 189). The 10-person, multidisciplinary commission was chaired by an attorney (Morris Abrams, professor of law, New York University) and began its work in 1980. [20] Compared to the *National Commission for the Protection of Human Subjects* its mandate was broader and not confined to ethical questions in research. It was invited to alter, or add to a list of issues. Like before, the commission studied the problems they addressed, listened to the specialists who helped them to think about the issues and withdrew in order to reflect on the questions from their own points of view. It then collaborated with the National Institute of Health's Office for Protection from Research Risks, and with the Food and Drug Administration in order to develop a guidebook for Institutional Review Boards. Based on the work that had been done in the 1960s and 1970s, the President's Commission identified consensus, disagreements and uncertainties. A model for finding consensus that could be reached on most of the topics (Ross 1986: 19–24). Their reasoning, agreements, uncertainties and disagreements were written in reports and during its three-year tenure, the commission held public readings throughout the country, commissioned research studies and published nine reports on "[...] medical-legal-ethical issues that seemed most pressing" (Ross 1986: 19). The reports provide practical decision-making policies, principles and guidelines. The most cited ones are: the *Definition of Death, Informed Consent, Deciding to Forego Life-Sustaining Treatment, Screening, Counselling for Genetic Conditions, Genetic Engineering* as well as *Access to Health Care*. The report *Deciding to Forego Life-Sustaining Treatment* (550 pages) is generally concerned with treatment decisions for incompetent patients. Permanently unconscious patients, seriously ill newborns as well as

---

20   Its original members were appointed by Jimmy Carter. The medical sociologist, Renee Fox, was one of the members.

decisions about cardiopulmonary resuscitation and Do-Not-Resuscitate (DNR) orders are discussed in particular. Besides an analysis of the problems, the report includes specific recommendations and conclusions about who should make decisions to forego treatment and how those decisions should be made (President's Commission 1983).

According to Renee Fox (1990), a number of these reports have had considerable influence on public opinion and public policy, medical and hospital practice as well as legislative action, and legal decision-making. Fox supposes that the Commission's volumes on *Defining Death* (July 1981), and *Deciding to Forego Life-Sustaining Treatment* (March 1983) have probably had the most influence (Fox 1990: 205). Influence on a judiciary level is also stated by Judith Ross: "[...] court decisions routinely cite these reports as authoritative statements on bioethics issues" (Ross 1986: 19). Although the Commission's recommendations did not have the force of a law, they were embraced by courts and legislature acted upon them. According to Ross, they were treated like an unwritten law (Ross 1986: 19).

The President's Commission concluded that in order to protect the interests of patients who lack decision-making capacity and to ensure their well-being and self-determination, health care staff along with administrators and trustees ought to explore and evaluate various formal and informal administrative arrangements for review and consultation, such as ethics committees, especially for decisions that have life-or-death consequences. The commissioners realized the ongoing ethical problems in these decisions and therefore suggested that hospitals themselves should work out procedures in order to enhance decision making for "incompetent patients". Hospital Ethics Committees were supposed to be a reasonable means of promoting decision-making processes. Ross recommends that Hospital Ethics Committees should be particularly familiar with the reports on (1) *Defining Death, and* (2) *Deciding to Forego Life-Sustaining Treatment* as well as (3) *Making Health Care Decisions,* and (4) *Security Access to Health Care* (Ross 1986: 19). In the second report named above, the President's Commission recommends four possible roles for Hospital Ethics Committees: (a) diagnostic and prognostic review; (b) staff education by providing forums for the discussion of ethical issues and methodological instruction in resolving ethical dilemmas; (c) institutional policy and guideline formulation with regard to specific ethical issues; (d) review of treatment decisions made by physicians, patients or surrogate; and (e) decision-making about specific cases. With respect to the educational task of Hospital Ethics Committees, the Commission stresses the importance of diverse membership and shared perspectives. The committee should "[...] serve as a focus for community discussion and educa-tion" (President's Commission 1983: 160–163). According to the President's Commission, courts should generally be used as decision-makers only as a last resort. The hope has been that Hospital Ethics Committees develop an ability to facilitate local, consensual decision making. Following Cranford, in which way and to what extent this hope has become true is difficult to ascertain (Ross 1986: 7).

Jonathan Moreno criticizes the President's Commission's remarks on ethics committees in *Deciding to Forego Life-Sustaining Treatment* for its ambiguous treatment of committees as advisory panels or as decision mak-ers (Moreno 1995: 100). On the one hand an advisory role is strongly sug-gested as an ethicist and member of a committee put forward that the one overriding theme of the meetings has been: "We make no decisions"; on the other hand the report goes on in favour for a more decisive role of Hospital Ethics Committees (President's Commission 1983: 163; Cranford, Doudera 1984: 13): Instead of having the doctor who takes complete responsibility for patients in these situations, it seems reasonable to ask an institutional body to represent and safeguard the patient's interests.

But, if the truly difficult issue was whether the court could dare to tell physicians how to treat, or not to treat their patients, then a clinical com-mittee instead could hardly please physicians (Ross 1986: 7). Moreno re-marks:

"My impression is that the Commission intended to allow the possibility that ethics committees could actually make decisions for specific patients when the only other option is going to court. [...] The most likely situation in which there would be a stark choice between a court and the ethics committee is that of a terminally ill and incapacitated patient lacking directives or a surrogate" (1995: 100).

What can be summed up at this point is, that there are no specific com-petencies defined for Hospital Ethics Committees. Mostly they deal with questions that concern issues of life-and-death. It turns out that not ques-tions of technology are central, but of living and dying. And finally, these forums are seen as an alternative to the court by offering quite a bit of pro-tection for physicians and the hospital.

In 1981, the President's Commission had initiated a national survey of Hospital Ethics Committees which revealed that less than 1 percent of American hospitals had ethics committees (President's Commission 1983: 443–446). However, Cranford and Doudera remark, that it should be noticed that Stuart Youngner and his colleagues, who did the study, utilized a very narrow definition of an ethics committee (Cranford, Doudera 1984: 14). While the President's Commission began supporting the building of Hospital Ethics Committees, yet, another regulatory impetus for the establishment of ethics committees appeared shortly after the Commission's reports: "The Baby Jane Doe and Baby Doe Cases".

From the "Baby Does' Cases" to Infant Bioethical Review Committees

In spring 1982, a child with "Down Syndrome" (Baby Jane Doe) with a malformed gullet (esophageal atresia) was born in Bloomington, Indiana. Some physicians recommended immediate surgical repair of the atresia while others thought that the infant's quality of life would not be good after treatment and therefore no operation should be offered. The baby should just be kept comfortable and be allowed to die. The parents decided for non-treatment and the hospital administration went to court to reverse the parents' decision. In between a series of court hearings, rulings, and appeals, the baby died of starvation. As long as it was recommended by a physician, Indiana judges affirmed the parent's right to choose non-treatment for the child (Cranford, Doudera 1984).

The case received widespread and mostly negative publicity. Public outcry was included in numerous newspapers, magazine articles and editorials, and a response to this highly publicized case, was federal government intervention: The Department of Health and Human Services (DHHS) published regulations on neonatal care (Cranford, Doudera 1984). Health care professionals asked themselves how to avoid federal intervention, and as a consequence, the American Academy of Pediatrics promulgated policy on critically ill newborns in response to the proposed "Baby Doe" governmental regulations that had been finally struck down in court (Moreno 1995: 81). The Academy included recommendations about the formation of *Infant Bioethical Review Committees* that the DHHS's final rule acknowledged and strongly encouraged, but did not mandate its use in hospitals caring for newborns (McCormick 1984: 150).

In fall 1983, a baby was born with spina bifida and hydrocephaly in New York ("the case of Baby Doe"). The parents decided for conservative treatment and refused surgery. Parents and physicians risked legal involvement when treatment decisions were made in these 'gray' areas, especially, when life-prolonging or aggressive treatment was withheld.

In this year (1983) the first national conference on Hospital Ethics Committees was held in Washington DC. According to Judith Randal, more than "200 doctors, hospital administrators, clergy, nurses, social workers, health planners, and others attended from thirty-eight states and Canada" (Randal 1983: 10). As Randal explains, the conference made clear that there is widespread interest in their future, but many difficulties will still remain (Randal 1983: 10). Problems about their composition, goals, functioning, scope of responsibility, mandate as well as financing were discussed (Rosner 1985: 2697). The typical committee was said to be chaired by a physician, "to be called into session infrequently, and then to meet on behalf of an incompetent and critically ill patient for whom there is little or no hope of recovery" (Rosner 1985: 2697). Whether decisions of ethics committees should be binding and whether an ethics committee should ever go to court to seek enforcement of its views belonged to the crucial questions being debated on (Rosner 1985: 2697). Another key issue that came up during the conference was whether Hospital Ethics Committees can be expected "to do better than physicians or the courts in resolving the ethical dilemmas that arise in applying technology to patient care" (Randal 1983: 10).

John Robertson, a University of Texas law professor describes three possible types of Hospital Ethics Committees (1984). "The optional-optional model" of HECs has as an educational and conscious-raising function for the institution by identifying areas where policy decisions may need to be made. According to Robertson, the committee should be prepared to help resolve disputes about care of the severely ill and should operate on a standby basis. Nevertheless, he remarks that the service should not be obligatory. He recommended that every hospital should at least establish the "optional-optional model" (Robertson 1984: 442–443). The alternatives, he outlines, are "mandatory" committees which would require physicians to meet committee members and follow their advice. His third suggestion is the alternative of a "mandatory-optional" ethics committee: Physicians would have to consult the committee when a critical decision is to be made, but would be free to ignore its recommendations if they choose (Robertson 1984: 443–444).

In the same year, the President's Commission cited a proposed model to establish Hospital Ethics Committees: The scope of authority of such committees would be to review treatment decisions made on behalf of "terminally ill incompetent patients, review treatment decisions made by terminally ill competent patients who request committee review, review medical decisions having ethical implications, provide counselling, establish guidelines, and educate" (Rosner 1985: 2696). The model bill also suggested multidisciplinary membership of nine persons appointed by the chief hospital administrators for one-year renewable terms. Moreover, the committee should be accessible to the staff of the hospital and patients, should convene within three days of a request, "keep minutes, arrive at a recommendation by majority vote, place a copy of its recommendation in the patient's hospital record, and provide a copy of the recommendation to the person who requested the committee's review of a treatment or other medical decision" (Rosner 1985: 2696).

Proponents of Hospital Ethics Committees first asserted that ethics committees would satisfy the need for a more systematic and principled approach to the contemporary dilemmas of medical as well as ethical decision-making within hospital and long-care facilities (Cranford, Doudera 1984: 15). Another benefit is seen in the committees' chance to serve as a link between societal values and the actual development occurring in the institutions that care for and treat particular patients who manifest ethical dilemmas (Cranford, Doudera 1984: 15). Finally, ethics committees, and the evolving network, will help to distinguish between ethical dilemmas where a consensus seems to exist and those where no consensus seems achievable. But, there are however:

"[…] many areas where consensus does not, at least at this time, exist. Two of these are treatment for handicapped newborns and the provision of fluids and nutrition to the hopelessly ill. Although ethics committees cannot resolve problems that lack societal agreement, those institutions having ethics committees are at least able to address such dilemmas in an open and constructive manner" (Cranford, Doudera 1984: 16).

Then in 1984, Federal Child Abuse Amendments plus the DHHS regulations required all States to have a mechanism for making sure that their intensive care nurseries were not engaging in discriminatory practices and recommended using *Infant Care Review Committees* to review decisions on forgoing life-saving treatment for newborns as a less intrusive alternative to federal investigation. At the national level, the American Hospital Association and the Catholic Hospital Association declared formal recommendation about Hospital Ethics Committees, seen as a potential means to ensure good decision-making practices. Finally, even the American Medical Association supported ethics committees (Ross 1986: 7).

By early 1985 one survey showed: Among hospitals with Neonatal Intensive Care Units (NICUs), more than half had ethics committees. A majority of teaching hospitals had ethics committees and it was found out that even hospitals without ethics committees were thinking about forming them. By size, only hospitals with 500 beds or more showed significant increases in ethics committees. Most commonly, administrators, nurses, and the clergy were found on the committees, followed by legal counsel, social workers, patient representatives, and philosopher ethicists. These committees facilitated decision-making by clarifying important issues, providing legal protection for hospital administration and staff, making consistent hospital policies, and providing a forum for the airing of professional disagreements (Cranford, Doudera 1984: 15).

The Catholic Health Association conducted a survey of its member institutions and found that 41 percent met its definition of an ethics committee (Kalchbrenner, Kelly, McCarthy 1983: 47). 19 percent reported committees that served for decision-making processes, and 17 percent that functioned as policy making groups. Among the surveyed hospitals, committees played an active role in recommending policies to all levels of the hospital organization. The use of DNR orders was identified as the most common area for policy recommendation, followed by policies on Living Wills and the withdrawal of treatment (Cranford, Doudera 1984). Cranford and Doudera resume:

"The President's Commission gave prominence to the idea of ethics committees at a fortuitous time. Although the bioethics community had been worrying about decisions to forego treatment for handicapped infants and terminally ill patients for many years, there had not been sufficient concern either within the health care industry or from the body politic to turn that concern into action. With the two Baby Doe cases (as well as a number of movies, television programs, and other popular treatments of these issues), the question jelled and many more ethics committees were formed" (Cranford, Doudera 1984: 13–14).

Considering nursing, the study by Youngner et al. (1983) also revealed that 57 percent of ethics committee members were physicians and that nurses were restricted: only 31 percent of committees allowed nurses to present cases and only 50 percent of the nurses were allowed to attend a meeting (Youngner et al. 1983: 443–449). It should be of concern if nurses, the largest group of health professionals, are not adequately represented in the committee. Moreover they are rather rarely invited to present cases which implies that there is no place in the institution to which they can turn for formal exploration of their perceived conflicts (see Relational Analysis, chapter three).

In 1984, the House of Delegates of the American Nurses' Association (ANA) had adopted the following with regard to nurses' participation in multidisciplinary institutional review: "[...] promote nurses' active participation in the development, implementation, and evaluation of formal mechanism for multidisciplinary institutional ethical review such as institutional ethics committees" (ANA, Code for Nurses with Interpretative Statements 1985).

In addition to court cases and government intervention, other conditions during the late 1970s and early 1980s fostered the belief that Hospital Ethics Committees could resolve new and complex health care ethical dilemmas. Firstly, the argument that new medical technology has been creating ethical situations persisted, and secondly, the argument was raised that patients and their relatives would no longer accept passive roles, but demanded an active part in making decisions about treatment. This anti-paternalistic position is reflected in the patient's rights movement, the development of informed consent as well as the growth of patient advocacy as a goal of nursing practice (see Relational Analysis, chapter three). It resulted in the assumption that each human being was an autonomous agent who is able of making decisions as long as being fully informed with regard to medical care and his or her life. Closely connected to this movement was the change of society's trust in physician's behaviour (Rothman 2003: 222). Sichel points to questions of mistrust about receiving excessive Medicare and Medicaid payments (Sichel 1992: 115). She thinks:

"[...] malpractice suits against hospitals and physicians have caused health care professionals and institutions considerable concern about how they might protect themselves (and) [...] time was ripe for a new structure for making medical ethical decision; an autonomous physician no longer could make all medical and ethical judgements for his or her patients" (1992: 116).

It seemed to be obvious that these decisions required a growing sensitivity. The answer was seen in improved education of the health care team as well as the parents about the "[...] practical implications of disabilities, specific hospital policies to assist the decision makers, and recognition that parents and doctors – those who held the legal responsibility for making these very difficult decisions – needed as much help as they could get in making the decision" (Ross 1986: 7).

Both the Department of Health and Human Services as well as the American Academy of Pediatrics strongly recommended that each hospital providing newborn care, especially the ones with Neonatal Intensive Care

Units (NICUs), should form *Infant Review Committees*. The recommendations given by the Academy of Pediatrics and the DHHS could add to the President's Commission statement which had endorsed the idea of ethics committees in general. Some State legislatures, hospitals and State medical associations as well as insurance companies passed resolutions that approved Hospital Ethics Committees.

On the whole, Cranford and Doudera are convinced that the most compelling impetus has been the regulations – first given by government and then by professional organizations – as reaction to the story of "Infant Doe", a case of non-treatment of a newborn with "Down Syndrome" (Cranford, Doudera 1984: 13). However, Cranford and Doudera remark that Hospital Ethics Committees were growing in a free-form way, with no requirements for representation, and no clear delimited tasks, or no set procedures. And yet: No formal mandate for coming into being (Cranford, Doudera 1984: 13). Following Ross, ethics committees were at a crucial point since they had been given institutional support as well as governmental encouragement, but, what they ought to do and the way they should do it has not been made precisely clear. Education, policy development and case review are said to be their potential functions. "They will need to define their own tasks carefully and to use their limited time and energy wisely [...] must be able to bend their differences to find consensus, and yet preserve those differences so that they do not become rubber stamps for a single point of view. [...]" (Ross 1986: 8).

To sum up, the development of contemporary Hospital Ethics Committees is marked by eventful stories: the Baby Doe Cases which raised questions about the "beginning of life" and the Karen Quinlan story that put, supported by media, the "end of life" debate forward, locally in hospitals as well as governmentally and publicly. As a result, the attention focused on ethics committees in the seventies can be traced to three sources. First, beginning in 1976, the ruling in the Karen Quinlan case by the New Jersey Supreme Court. Second, in its report, *Deciding to Forego Treatment*, the President's Commission for the Study of *Ethical Problems in Medicine and Biomedical and Behavioural Research* discussed the potential for, and advocated the further research into Hospital Ethics Committees. Finally, the American Academy of Pediatrics responded to the "Baby Doe" regulations which were issued by the United States Department of Health and Human Services by proposing the formation of *Infant Bioethical Review Committees*. As a consequence, the DHHS' final rule acknowledged this idea and endorsed the use of *Infant Care Review Committees*.

Statutory Authority for Hospital Ethics Committees, Bureaucratization and Evaluation

Although not very much referred to in literature, it is noteworthy that the impetus for ethics committees in the years following the court cases came not only from government but also from the self-regulation of the health care industry: mainly in connection with "quality assurance".

A 1992 action by the Joint Commission for the Accreditation of Health-care Organizations (JCAHO) formalized the institutionalization of clinical ethics. For accreditation, hospitals and other health care institutions were required to have in place "mechanism(s) for the consideration of ethical issues arising in the care of patients" and to provide education to caregivers and patients on ethical issues in health care (JCAHO 1992: 105). Although Hospital Ethics Committees were not clearly and explicitly mentioned, they became the favored way for institutions to respond to these various new guidelines and requirements. This mandate to create an ethics case review process motivated the professional hospital community to look at the quality of its practice (Tulsky, Fox 1996).

New York as a State that is orientated towards activism and regulation, requires ethics committees of every hospital and nursing home. Moreover, there are more recommendations put forward by the *Governor's Task Force on Life and the Law* being concerned with decision making on behalf of incapacitated patients without advance directives or a durable power of attorney for health care (Moreno 1995: 102).

In 1992 the task force proposed that family members or close friends should be recognized in the law as surrogates for patients. "To provide some public assurance and accountability that surrogates are acting in good faith, all decisions to forego life-sustaining treatment for non-dying patients would be subject to retrospective review by a facility-based 'bioethics committee'" (Moreno 1995: 102). The structure as well as general procedures including multidisciplinary membership were also set forth in the bill. If patients do not have a surrogate, the ethics committee itself can make decisions concerning the termination of life-sustaining treatment (Moreno 1995: 102). New York legislation specified two ethical standards that surrogates and ethics committees are supposed to follow: Decisions have to be made either according to the wishes of the patient, or if they cannot be known, in his or her best interest (Moreno 1995: 102).

With the New York proposal the history of ethics committees has reached the point of legally required procedural decision making in the clinical setting. The task force hoped that bioethics committees would become accepted in analogy to Institutional Review Boards (Moreno 1995: 103). "Once created by the medical profession as a consultative mechanism composed entirely of physicians, committees that took a role in clinical ethics review have gradually acquired more regulatory authority [...]" (Moreno 1995: 103).

On the whole, most of the information about ethics committees came from an initial nationwide survey of hospital ethics committees, and from follow-up surveys focusing on particular regions or specific occupations. Despite the surveys, there was a need for more information about ethics committees, their composition, and how the members attained their membership (Tulsky, Fox 1996). Nurses expressed continuing concern for adequate representation on and access to ethics committees to discuss patient care situations and policies (Aroskar 1984). What can be said about their tasks and functions at this point?

Jonathan Moreno argues that there might be no interesting difference between an ethics committee and any other bureaucratic entity in a complex social structure such as a hospital (Moreno 1995: 91). In the sense that committees represent bureaucratic lines of authority and control, all committees can be seen as political entities. Its multidisciplinary membership, its procedures, or its political or legal functions are all quite similar to those of other committees. Owing to their inherently political nature, committees could include reflections of established powers and poor sites for resolving an institution's moral quandaries (Lo 1987). As pointed out before, Betty Sichel is convinced: "No matter what articles about IECs state, a primary purpose for these committees is to protect health care institutions and personnel against malpractice claims" (Sichel 1992: 116). Based on her analysis, she regards the emphasis on the legal consequences of health care policy and medical decisions as one possible reason for arguing that a principled "ethics of justice and rights" underlies deliberations of Clinical Ethics Committees (Sichel 1992: 116). According to Sichel, a second reason for applying a theory of justice to the deliberations of Hospital Ethics Committees "[...] is that certain policies and decisions involve questions of competition, prioritization, and scarce resources" (Sichel 1992: 116). She concludes: "Such a committee might justify the unequal allocation of scarce resources, provided that ethical principles govern the procedures, deliberation, and decisions on the distribution of these resources and the making of medical policy about such distribution" (Sichel 1992: 116).

The actual work of many of these bodies does not always consist of helping resolve ethical disputes as a moral philosopher or theologian understands the concept. "Indeed, addressing communication problems, searching for additional facts, or uncovering medico-legal misconceptions are among the activities typical of ethics committees" (Moreno 1995: 92). In fact, most committees stress "advisory" rather than a "decision-making" capacity. They regard their functions as mediation and the improvement of communication (Moreno 1995: 92).

Then, the American Society for Bioethics Consultation together with the American Society for Health and Human Values responded by creating a joint task force to explore standards for ethics consultation. After two years of meeting, drafting and revising documents, the result, *Core Competencies for Health Care Ethics Consultation* was published in 1998 by the American Society for Bioethics and Humanities (ASBH)[21] that aroused interest beyond the bioethics community (Aulisio, Arnold, Youngner 1999). Nevertheless, each institution experienced limitations of general guidelines, and had to face different problems in building up committees (Lo 2003) as also pointed out by Ronald Cranford in the following.

In 2003, on the first international assessment summit on Hospital Ethics Committees, Cranford who has been watching the development of ethics consultation in the United States declares it to be "[…] a movement to be […] still in its earliest stages, where there is still no high consensus on many major aspects […]" (Cranford 2002: 1). According to Cranford there had been three extremes: First, the 'medical model' e.g. prognosis committees; second, the pure ethics model, which emphasized education on the ethical principles relevant to an individual case; third, a process model, focused on sound decision making practices at the bedside (Cranford 2002: 1). For him, the most controversial issues are DNR, brain death, nutrition and hydration (Cranford 2002: 1). What are the main objections to and problems of ethics committees being discussed?

"One of the largest problems is physicians' resistance. It is well known that many physicians are indifferent to, and frequently hostile to, what they regard as the 'intrusion' of ethics on their turf" (McCormick 1984: 153). However, a study published in 1991 reveals that physicians are not opposed

---

21 ASBH is the successor to the Society for Health and Human Values (SHHV), the Society for Bioethics Consultation (SBC), and the American Association of Bioethics (AAB).

to the establishment of ethics committees, that is to say, nearly nine of ten physicians believed ethics committees were needed in hospitals (Finkenbine, Gramelspacher 1991). In which way are they themselves served? One study finding is: In 78 percent of the cases discussed in Hospital Ethics Committees, recommendations are made to the medical staff; in 62.5 percent they are also made to the hospital board and in 48 percent to the nursing department. The greatest number of policies have been developed around the issues of resuscitation (94 percent), Living Wills (53 percent) and the withdrawal of treatment (50 percent) (Oddi; Cassidy 1990).

Most evaluations of clinical ethics committees have been concerned with developing or improving specific Hospital Ethics Committee programs, "often on the basis of narrow internal criteria (e.g. outcomes), not with assessing whether the programs fulfill broader criteria such as those contained in the recommendations of the President's Commission" (McBurney 2001: 180). Of course, evaluating the policy and educational initiatives of Hospital Ethics Committees can reveal who participated in their creation and implementation, but that kind of evaluation is not likely to answer questions about who is not being invited to an "ethics" committee, whose voices are not being heard, and what the reasons for an exclusion are. Those questions are asked in the contextual study by Janet Storch and Glenn Griener (1992), Cate McBurney refers to in her article *Ethics Committees and Social Change. Plus ca change?*

"By excavating the social, political, economic, and cultural milieux within which ICE's operate, contextual analysis can help find answers to these questions. And those answers could help to determine whether IECs are a genuine alternative to the judical or governmental processes to which people traditionally turn when they are not being heard" (2001: 181).

Storch and Griener could show how the interdisciplinary consultation was seen as an important support service to physicians by hospital administrators. Ethics committees were *not* seen as a support to nurses. The overall impression the researchers gained from their interviews is that administrators support these committees but may have a relatively narrow perception of its role. "Perhaps, many of these hospital administrators see such committees as a 'nice to have' because it seems that ethical issues are being attended to in the hospital, thereby reassuring the administrator and the board and serving as a symbol to staff and the general public" (Storch, Griener 1992: 25).

The Talk and its Performance in Hospital Ethics Committees

In the early 1990s questions about the work of and in Hospital Ethics Committees were raised with an attention to context, narrative, and power relationships. Susan Rubin and Laurie Zoloth-Dorfman state:

"In a world of talk, where the hearers and tellers of narrative [...] and the ethics committees all serve as an answering chorus, we need to pay close attention not only to what is said, but to who talks, who listens, and how – we need to 'see' the 'talk', and the performance of the 'talk', as clearly as we study the substance of the argument" (Zoloth-Dorfman 1996: 321).

Rubin and Zoloth-Dorfman found out that of all the power relationships among health care professionals in the clinical setting "the gendered relationship is one of the most fundamental" (Zoloth-Dorfman 1996: 321), and that this also accounts for the talk in Hospital Ethics Committees. In their words "gender approximates power" (Zoloth-Dorfman 1996: 322), and these "power differentials are potentiated by a cultural valence that surrounds and is reified by such gender-specific roles as 'nurse' (overwhelmingly female) and 'social' worker (overwhelmingly female)" (Zoloth-Dorfman 1996: 322). They state that it is the directive authority of the physician that is central in the clinical setting, "and the cleaning, soothing, feeding, and teaching that is nursing [...]" (Zoloth-Dorfman 1996: 322).

Also based on their linguistic literature review, Rubin and Zoloth-Dorfman come to say that men tend to be more concerned than women with their own status in the interaction, "hence their focus on avoiding a 'one down' position and their comfort asserting confidently their views, even if they have doubts about them" (Zoloth-Dorfman 1996: 325). Linguistic analysis of power relations have shown that the use of indirect communication is associated strongly with persons of relatively less power and authority (Zoloth-Dorfman 1996: 325). Whose voices are most heard and valued in discussing issues of concern in patient care is dependent on the hierarchical setting like a hospital: Profession, rank, and degree often determine the extent to which permission is given to speak freely and authoritatively (Zoloth-Dorfman 1996: 327). Rubin and Laurie Zoloth-Dorfman point out that those who are perceived to have "the most authority and expertise, those with the strongest opinions, those with the most assertive speaking style, those who talk the loudest, or those who simply talk the most have enormous power in shaping and controlling the discussion [...] women are disproportionately represented in the categories that speak and are heard less" (Zoloth-Dorfman 1996: 327).

As Virginia Warren (1992) had found out, the authors add that women tend to occupy less verbal space in conversations, and need greater and often specific encouragement to speak their opinions aloud. Reflecting on the meaning and significance of asking questions or raising concerns, for the authors it is clear, that what is at stake, particularly for those with less power and experience, is reputation. With regard to nurses Zoloth-Dorfman observed:

"Therefore, we have found that many staff nurses are more likely to publicly hide their ethical concerns out of fear of reprisal, or, as they tell us, fear of developing a reputation of being 'difficult'. [...] When we hear that asking questions, voicing concerns, or raising objections are not considered safe or acceptable, we are concerned about the decline of independent moral agency, professional responsibility, and personal integrity" (Zoloth-Dorfman 1996: 327).

Looking at *naming*, that is to say, how ethics committee members address each other, Rubin and Laurie Zoloth-Dorfman observed that it is not uncommon, even between long-time colleagues, to hear the female nurse of the ethics committee refer to and address the male physician as "Dr. X" and to have him respond to her and refer to her by her first name (Zoloth-Dorfman 1996: 328).

Virginia Warren takes into consideration that moral questions are often formulated in a competitive way. For example, questions of decision-making for "not-capacitated" patients would be often framed in terms of who decides for the patients. The debate then, she remarks, is over the question of authority (Warren 1992: 36–38). She also suggests that important features of the moral context are obscured by appeals for neutrality. By stressing the value of neutrality, the particular features of the situation would often be ignored. For her, the dominant trend in philosophical ethics has been to regard people as best able to decide what is moral when least tied to place and time and when least connected through ties or partiality to family and community (Warren 1992: 36–38). This practice of abstracting oneself from the particularities produces two kinds of distortions: First, it denies consideration of those experiences that shape how an agent perceives her or his role in a situation. "By substracting those features that shed light on their experience and life, such individuals may become, at least in part, invisible to themselves" (Warren 1992: 33). Second, distortion arises from the creation of and emphasis on a picture of "generic persons and relationships" (Warren 1992: 33). Hence, it is likely to lose important factors about psychological well-being, as well as other facets of character that bear on a particular situation or potential resolution.

With more focus on how case discussions are framed in Hospital Ethics Committees Flynn observed that the speakers have been more concerned with ethical principles than the processes by which decisions can be reached. Negotiation took place, but there were not equal resources or equal power relationships in the organization or in the committee meetings (Flynn 1991a: 183). In her field research, Flynn found out that there is a pattern of talk in Hospital Ethics Committees, when

"[...] dealt with ethics at all was to present the case, and then someone would say: 'What is the ethical principle?' and another person, often the ethicist, would say, as in a mantra, 'autonomy' or 'allocation of resources'. The incantations of justice, autonomy, beneficence, non-maleficence, veracity, and fidelity were heard throughout the committees. In one committee, the chair would press for two ethical principles that were in conflict, so that the response might be, for example: 'autonomy' and he would ask 'versus?' and someone would sing out 'justice'" (Flynn 1991a: 182).

Here, a very instrumental use of principles evolves. One can doubt that this model of consultation might augment the machinery of ethical principles in shaping perceptions. Margaret Urban Walker critically asks:

"Aren't abstract principles often given (sometimes new) meaning under the impact of concrete cases, rather than cases being simply 'decided' by the 'application' of principles? And who or what decides what is a 'case' – a moral problem – in the first place, as well what sort of case-subject to what principle or principles – it is?" (Walker 1993: 34).

John Evans sees the use of principles as a method that takes the complexity of actually lived moral life and translates this information into scales by discarding information that resists translation and thus creates a language that brings order to difficult problems (Evans 2000: 32–34). He thinks that the principles were created to "enhance calculability and simplify bioethical decision-making" (Evans 2000: 32).

Walker opposes against the use of principles to simplify decision-making. She is convinced about the idea that "a story, or better, *history* is the basic form of representation for moral problems" (Walker 1993: 35). Therefore, she suggests that it is necessary to know "who the parties are, how they understand themselves and each other, what terms of relationship have brought them to this [...] problematic point, and perhaps what social or institutional frames shape or circumscribe their options" (Walker 1993: 35). She states:

"If moral accounts must make sense to those by whom, to whom, and about whom they are given, the integrity of these accounts is compromised when some parties to a moral situation are not heard or respresented. If chances are missed for different perspectives that open critical opportunities, moral community is doubly ill served, alternate narratives go unexplored, and some members are in practice disqualified as agents of value" (Walker 1993: 37).

In sum, the use of principles in Hospital Ethics Committees needs critical consideration. It sounds like an engineering model that supports a way of dealing with "cases" and framing questions in a technical way. Hereby, narratives that show the context of a specific situation might get excluded or issues of conflict and concern that do not fit the principle-model can be marginalized.

The German Development:
A Re-Make of the US-American Model

The implementation of Hospital Ethics Committees in Germany after the US-American model of the 1980s has been favoured from its inception and is still supported by leading organizations with regard to ethics in healthcare. For example, the Academy for Ethics in Medicine (AEM) serves as an advisory body for clinical practice and education. The establishment of Hospital Ethics Committees has constantly been put in a bright light in publications, speeches and flyers (Simon, 2000; Neitzke 2002; May 2004; Vollmann, Wernstedt 2005). Publications about Hospital Ethics Committees start with a historical flashback situated in the USA when in 1976 the New Jersey Supreme Court decided In the Matter of Karen Quinlan, in which physician and the family struggled for authority of medical decision in the case of a persistently unconscious patient. There have not yet been critical writings that put the establishment of Hospital Ethics Committees into question. On the contrary, within current critiques on economization processes in German Health Care, Hospital Ethics Committees are rather seen as critical forums themselves.

The Center for Ethics in Health Care *(Zentrum für Gesundheitsethik – ZfG)* at the Lutheran Academy Loccum is especially active in offering educational classes on the establishment and inner workings of hospital ethics committees. The educators are philosophers, medical doctors, and theologians. Some of them were not only convinced by the model academically, but they got to know it by visiting the States. They are the same persons who have published most of the German articles on hospital ethics committees (Simon, 2000; Neitzke 2002; May 2004; Vollmann, Wernstedt 2005). All publications refer to the US-American model of Hospital Ethics Committees of the 1980s and describe the three functions: Education, policy development and case consultation. With regard to historical events, some texts mention that the starting point of Hospital Ethics Committees traces back to the US-American case-story of Karen Quinlan.

The following historical steps of German hospital ethics committees show some similarity with the historical steps of US-American contemporary Hospital Ethics Committees: (1) When the first Hospital Ethics Committees were established in 1997, the German Lutheran and Catholic Church Association published a joint recommendation brochure to establish such committees, explicitly according to the US-American model (Deutscher Evangelischer Krankenhausverband, Katholischer Krankenhausverband 1997). In 2000 a survey revealed that among 795 members of the Christian Churches' Association, 30 hospitals declared to have an ethics committee or a comparable arrangement to offer consultation (Simon, Gillen 2000). (2) Along with the installation of quality management instruments and since the Accreditation Organizations of Health Care have demanded that hospitals should have policies and procedures to cope with ethical issues, the number of institutions which declare to have Hospital Ethics Committees has been growing fast (Kettner, May 2002). (3) The German Physicians' Association has published a call to establish Hospital Ethics Committees. A diversity in structure and practices is explained by a lack of standards and the individual histories of the hospitals. The physicians' Association strongly recommends to establish a standard as soon as possible (Wiesing 2006).

According to an analysis by the philospher Matthias Kettner (2005), Hospital Ethics Committees serve as a helpful instrument to meet a so-called "moral insecurity" due to technological progress and a plurality of values, not only among professionals at the bedside, but also among people in public.

Moreover, I think, Hospital Ethics Committees can offer new jobs for philosophers and are establishing a market place for medical ethicists who are selling more and more classes on applied ethics. Thereby their own ideas, concepts, and interests that serve their status quo (in medicine, philosophy and law) are stabilized.

On the whole, I resume, rather than being a space for reflecting conflicts and being a voice of critique, Hospital Ethics Committees tend to develop as a form of regulatory ethics that allow a more powerful internal role in organized medicine. While these committees are rapidly growing in Germany, the following questions have been left open: What are the criteria for a good practice in clinical ethics committees and who is going to define it? Questions such as what these committees are actually doing, who they are serving, what issues they are addressing, in which way they are accessed, and the degree of satisfaction of the users of the service have not been empirically addressed yet.

4 Summary

Hospital Ethics Committees arguably had their roots in kidney-dialysis selection committees and can be traced back even further. As recently as the early 1980s, Hospital Ethics Committees were a relatively rare phenomenon as national surveys estimated that they were present in fewer than one percent of US-American hospitals. Ethical considerations were limited to oversee research and took place in Institutional Review Boards (IRBs). During the 1980s, Hospital Ethics Committees began to grow rapidly in response to such "cases" as those involving Karen Quinlan and Baby Doe, as well as to the 1983 report of the President's Commission for the Study of Ethical Problems in Medicine. Consequently, the number of Hospital Ethics Committees grew, in less than a decade, to more than 60 percent. Nowadays, in the United States, every health care institution has at least one, but often several ethics committees that is largely the result of the Joint Commission on the Accreditation of Healthcare Organization's (JCAHO's) 1992 mandate. German proponents of Hospital Ethics Committees, mostly medical ethicists have started what I identified as a re-make of the US-American model of these committees. By retelling the contemporary development of US-Hospital Ethics Committees as a linear history of success and a necessity due to technological progress, Germany has taken up the idea that these committees should serve as a link between societal values and the actual developments occurring in the institutions that care for and treat patients. As once in the United States, the rapid growth of Hospital Ethics Committees had been caused by the Joint Commission on the Accreditation of Health Care that demanded to have some structure available to meet ethical questions in hospitals; a similar development takes place in Germany: Accreditation is speeding up the number of HECs.

The analysis of the historical background reveals that the emergence of Hospital Ethics Committees cannot be reduced to reasons of technological progress. These institutionalized local committees in the United States are embedded within and have taken the direction from the emergent discipline of bioethics. They are a product of the complex interplay of events and governmental interventions. "In the case of Karen Quinlan" the court put significant power in the hands of the Hospital Ethics Committee which was specifically charged with making a medical determination that confirmed the attending physician's prognosis that Quinlan would not return to a "cognitive state". This is clearly a medical or clinical function and not an ethical one. The President's Commission emphasized that consultation and decision-making were a responsibility of the institution and they felt that Hospital Ethics Committees were one way to encourage institutions and staff to develop the practices of consultation and decision-making. The department of Health and Human Services said in the "Infant Doe" Regulations that Hospital Ethics Committees can bring about informed and fair decision making regarding difficult issues.

Throughout its history, the US-American ethics committee movement has been a topic of controversy. While proponents have seen such committees as a promising means of enhancing ethical decision making, possibly improving the quality of patient care, and protecting patients' rights; there are arguments given that they are little more than a shield to protect hospitals from litigation. Critics have also argued that such committees threaten to bureaucratize medical practice and that they build up an obstacle to the physician-patient relationship. Nevertheless, events like the invention of Kidney Dialysis Selection Committees and the building of a Multidisciplinary Advisory Committees as Prognosis Committees, revealed an increasingly interested public the insufficiency of internal professional norms to adequately govern medical practice.

As I could demonstrate, the support of Hospital Ethics Committees was after all an attempt to deal with developing problems of justice and prevent law suits. Thus, it served the institution of the hospital and physicians could find some sort of protections.

As studies on the work of Hospital Ethics Committees could show, Ruth Purtilo brought up when I interviewed her, and as I exemplified by the "Optimum Care Committee" in Boston Massachusetts General Hospital, questions about living and dying – like how to formulate Do Not Resuscitate orders – were dominating committee discussions. The theoretical framework of Hospital Ethics Committees' case discussions was principle-based. The tetrad of principles (autonomy, beneficence, non-maleficience and justice) promised relatively specific guidelines and proved to be more specific and objective than the previous Hippocratic ethic. The use of principles helped to work on calculations and a simplification of bioethical decision-making processes. Instead, especially feminist studies highlighted the importance of narrative and history to be the basic form of representation for moral problems.

Within the framework of *Situational Analysis,* I will now turn to the questions: "What social worlds are not present and active? Are there any worlds absent that I expected? Are there any surprising silences in the discourse?" (Clarke 2005: 115). In the world of bioethics and Hospital Ethics Committees, the social world of relatedness and dependency is a minor planet. Furthermore, while physicians in the role of 'final decision-makers' played an active role in the development of Hospital Ethics Committees, the role of nurses as the primary 'care-takers' of the patient – when the decision is made – is not part of the debate. I will now investigate into the notion of caring as a practice, the development of an "ethics of care" and the role of nurses.

Relational Analysis
Care and Hospital Ethics Committees

1 The Care Ethics Debate and Nursing since 1980

Care ethics can offer a perspective which is different from dominant ethical theories that have been criticized for being based too much on principles and for neglecting moral contexts embedded in social practices and historical settings. It emphasizes the importance of relatedness and difference to autonomy and consensus.

Compared to Germany, in the USA the literature about caring and nursing is huge, and its criticism no less. But, rather than analyze the myriad ways on how care can be defined, is understood, used, in which way it relates to nursing, and what the critique is, this chapter acknowledges the historical steps by tracing back the development of caring ideas. I focused on those that have first, mostly been discussed; second, have shaped the development of the care ethics debate from a nursing perspective and have third, fostered the development of "nursing ethics". Hereby, I have identified in what kind of discursive context each concept of care evolved and identified it as a kind of counter-argument like the "Care against Justice" or the "Touch against Technology" Debate. The aim is to shed light on the development of these counter-arguments from different perspectives of nursing and not to discuss what is "right" and what is "wrong", a "weak", or a "strong" argument to give rise to the importance of care practices. With regard to a nursing perspective the leading question is: What ideas were relevant to and used by nursing as a growing academic discipline with an increasing interest in ethics at that time?

Caring as a Women orientated Ethics and a Feminine Model

Being born, life starts in dependency, and in order to grow and develop, care is needed. And, at least in some parts of the life as an adult, all humans need to be cared for. Care work is needed for the sick, handicapped, frail elderly, and dying people. Susan Reverby (1987) has named this work "women's work" while Sara Ruddick has termed it as "caring labor" (1989). Care has been traditionally gendered in so far as most of the caring professions and care work, paid and unpaid, are practiced by women. Although care work is partly done professionally, the vast part is done privately.

Nurses have taken an interest in an "ethics of care" because it would capture their moral experiences better than a "male" "ethics of justice." As pointed out before, the historically embedded growth of an "ethics of care" are of interest here and not so much the philosophical underpinnings of the concepts themselves.

Caring as a Different Voice: Gilligan versus Kohlberg – Care versus Justice

Caring as it relates to ethics is rooted in the so called "Gilligan against Kohlberg" debate. What was the conflict about?

The late Harvard psychologist, Lawrence Kohlberg (1981) divided the moral development of individuals into three stages and claimed that people become morally mature by going through certain distinct stages. Being a mature adult, Kohlberg declares, you would have presumably outgrown the idea that "being good" would mean helping and pleasing other people (stage three on Kohlberg's scale). Then, you will have come to see that moral-ity consists of a set of rules for maintaining the social order (stage four). Furthermore, you could become even more mature to sum up the rules in a principle such as "the greatest good for the greatest number" (stage five), or to think of morality in terms of self-chosen universal principles of justice (stage six). Though, Kohlberg grants that not everyone reaches these levels of maturity. He found girls in comparison to boys not being able to make moral *judgements in terms of justice*. Thus, he declared them *not* to reach the last stage of moral reasoning (Kohlberg 1981).

Gilligan's book *In a different voice* (1982) motivated to ask for a *women oriented* ethics. In her view, human beings live their life in a *network of care and dependence*. Gilligan contrasted the *voice of care* with the *voice of justice*. Her research was designed in part as a corrective to the study on moral development by Lawrence Kohlberg. While Kohlberg had focused on boys, Gilligan instead focused on girls and in her empirical work she exclusively interviewed women. Rather than talking about rights and rules, these women were using the language of relationships and connection. They revealed the relevance of a contextual understanding and a look at concrete situations. According to this view, caring is seen as a moral orientation that gives an opportunity to see the particularities of the individual and relations as an integral part of moral judgement. Gilligan believes that impartiality fosters detachment which might breed moral blindness or indifference. Moreover, she points out, detachment might contribute to a failure to discern or *respond to* needs (Gilligan 1982). Gilligan is convinced that the aim of caring is not necessarily an agreement but mostly a *"shared understanding"* (Gilligan 1982).

Although her work deserves to be acknowledged for its relevance of keeping gender questions in mind and considering the limits of abstract principles in ethics, the methodological problem cannot be overseen: While Kohlberg has focused on boys, Gilligan has focused on girls and women. Thus, the studies are circumscribed by being male or female. The dichotomy of a "male ethics of justice" and a "female ethics of care" has not been overcome yet. A question that arises is whether there might not well be a feminine ethics of justice and / or a masculine ethics of care. For the further parts of my work here, I would also like to put into question, whether these distinctions are helpful to conceptualize care as a practice.

Caring as a Feminine Approach to Ethics:
Principle-based versus the Context-related

In her book *Caring. A Feminine Approach to Ethics and Moral Education* (1984), Nel Noddings argues that philosophy acknowledges basically the difference between pure and practical reason, but that ethics is treated in analogy with geometry: the focus is a set up of principles and logical deductions. In her view, ethics as the philosophical reflection on morality has too much concentrated on questions of moral foundation and judgement. She criticizes a moral judgement that is basically lead by abstract principles. Instead, she argues for a discussion on moral problems in terms of concrete situations which implies an "[...] approach of moral problems not as intellectual problems to be solved by abstract reasoning but as concrete human problems to be lived and to be solved in living" (Noddings 1984: 96). And this approach, as Noddings explains, is founded in "caring" (1984: 96).

The approach to ethics advocated by Noddings does not wholly ignore the theoretical contributions of traditional ethics but assumes that only certain aspects of these ethics can inform and enrich the moral life of the one who cares for others. Although her paradigm of a caring relation is the *mother-and-child dyad* and she moreover talks about a *feminine morality*. Nevertheless she remarks: "Both men and women may participate in the 'feminine' as I am developing it, but women have suffered acutely from its lack of explication" (Noddings 1984: 44).

Noddings emphasizes the importance of responsiveness to the needs of others that will contribute to better patient educational practice. Moreover, she renders meaning to the uniqueness of particular others and to the understanding of concrete situations. For her, caring is not so much a matter of actions, special tasks or processes as a mode of disposition, a virtue or a stance towards the other. For Noddings, caring is neither a principle nor a virtue in itself but it is based on relationships and there are no decisions that can be separated from their *contextual situation*. Caring gives rise to the development and exercise of virtues and for Noddings these must be assessed in the context of caring situations. She explains: "It is not, for example, patience itself that is a virtue but patience with respect to some infirmity or a particular cared-for or patience with respect to some infirmity of a particular cared-for or patience in instructing a concrete cared-for that is virtuous" (Noddings 1984: 96).

For Noddings, institutionalized care is destructive because it contradicts the *nature of care*. She thinks that a practice of care should be minimally regulated by standards and rather continuously be interpreted and shaped in the light of individual contexts.

"The duty to enhance the ethical ideal, the commitment to caring, invokes a duty to promote scepticism and non-institutional affiliation. In a deep sense, no institution or nation can be ethical. It cannot meet the other as one-caring or as one trying to care. It can only capture in general terms what particular ones-caring would like to have done in well-described situations. [...] Everything depends, then, upon the will to be good, to remain in caring relation to each other. How may we help ourselves and each other to sustain this will?" (1984: 103).

Particularly, Hilde Lindemann Nelson has criticized Nel Noddings' concept of care with regard to professional nursing (1992). For Noddings it has been central that the self-care of carers leads to a better care of others. Nelson criticizes that if the carers are so much devoted to someone else that

even their self-care is done as a service for others, thus, there is the danger
of fusion: "She (the carer) has identified her own interests and projects so
closely with those of the person for whom she cares that she stands in danger
of losing herself altogether" (Nelson 1992: 11). Hilde Lindemann Nelson
and Alisa Carse (1996) emphasize that the danger of exploitation threatens
care givers und therefore there should be set limits of having a duty to care
for others (1996: 19). Thereby, not only the danger of exploitation of care-
givers needs to be considered but also the danger that the ones being cared
for might be oppressed: "The need to set limits on care is an important
problem for the care ethic not only because of the danger of exploitation,
but also because of the danger of oppressing the recipient of care" (Carse,
Lindemann Nelson 1996: 22).[22]

Caring as a Foundational Concept for
a Theory of Nursing Ethics

In US-American nursing literature it is the notion of "caring" that is mostly
used to describe the work of nursing in relation to the patient. It is the
central term in nurses' definition of themselves and it is also the key notion
practicing nurses believe is their task. Nursing scholars like Patricia Benner
and Judith Wrubel use it in the title or subtitle of their books. Based on his
ten years of participant observations in hospitals, Daniel Chambliss points
out, that caring with regard to nursing is not seldomly used as a weapon in
their conflicts with physicians in order to distinguish between which nurses
do, that is "care" from what doctors do, which is "cure". Thereby nurses
put themselves in a morally superior position. When nurses say they "care",
this is not just a mere description of engaged practice, but a defence of their
importance (Chambliss 1996: 68).

Altogether, besides the monograph by Patricia Benner and Judith Wrubel (1989), there are mostly articles in US-American nursing journals that
give arguments and counter-arguments for an understanding of nursing
that involves a concept of care (Bishop, Scudder 1990). Some nursing scientists have explicitly outlined the significance of care within their theory of

---

22 In Germany, see Herta Nagl-Docekal and Herlinde Pauer-Studer (1993) as well as Gun-
    hild Buse (1993) and Carola Brucker (1990) who joined into the debate about care eth-
    ics.

nursing (Watson 1988) or have shown its meaning on the basis of empirical studies (Benner, Wrubel 1989, Benner 1994 a, b).

The following overview is based on a selection of those nursing ideas that have made caring to be the central thought for an understanding of nursing and those ideas that have put caring within the realm of nursing ethics.

Caring as a Protection of Human Dignity:
Care versus Cure – Touch versus Technology

It has frequently been noted that the difference between medicine and nursing is the difference between "curing" and "caring". Sally Gadow (1985) has articulated her observations as a nursing scientist and philosopher:

"The spectacular rise of technology in health care has cast a shadow on the image of caring, especially caring that is posited as the essence of a professional relationship. Caring has connotations like that of hospice, that is, taking care that patients are not abandoned when hope of cure is abandoned. While hope remains, however, it is not caring that will achieve cure; it is the technical expertise that repairs the valve or adjusts the dialysis. [...] Caring, while making patients feel more comfortable, perhaps even cherished, will not arrest pathology; thus it is not allowed to divert time and energy that can be invested in cure. Where there is no conflict between the two, it is because cure is impossible. When conflict arises, cure has priority" (Gadow 1985: 31).

For her, caring entails a commitment to a particular end, and that end, she proposes, is the protection of human dignity. According to Gadow, the reason, that technology poses a greater threat to dignity than does less complex care is related to what she calls the experience of otherness. She explains that mundane care as well as simple apparatus involve measures that persons usually can manage for themselves. "But complicated measures and machinery are more disruptive; they can remove the locus of control and of meaning from the individual by imposing otherness in two forms, the machine and the professional" (Gadow 1985: 36). First, the apparatus asserts an otherness that cannot be ignored or easily integrated into the physical or psychological being and second, complex techniques require greater expertise than many persons possess and professionals may be called to manage a procedure. Gadow resumes, that both elements of otherness, the apparatus as well as the expert, threaten to disrupt personal integrity, and thus violate dignity by removing patients from the center of their experience (Gadow 1985: 36). In addition, she states,

"[...] the domination by apparatus and by experts that can accompany the use of technology, patients can be reduced to objects in a more fundamental way than by the use of machines: in the view of the body as a machine. Such reduction occurs because regard for the body exclusively as a scientific object negates the validity of subjective meanings of the person's experience" (Gadow 1985: 36).

Gadow consequently asks: "Now that technology displays so vividly the reduction of persons to their objectness, what are the alternatives?" (Gadow 1985: 36). For her, two approaches suggest themselves as means of affirming the integrity of patients, one having to do with *truth*, and the other one with *touch*. She argues that disclosure can have a paternalistic basis. When patients are informed about their therapeutic value, irrespective of their wishes, she says that they would be addressed as objects and disclosure practices would also express a view of patients as objects since "[...] the belief that the truth to be disclosed (or withheld) is constituted entirely on the side of the caregiver, consisting of objective information, statistically ordered if possible" (Gadow 1985: 38). For her, those views imply that the "truth" of a situation exists independently of the persons involved. On the contrary, Gadow offers a view of "truth" as the most comprehensive and most personally meaningful interpretation of the situation possible. She remarks: "The opposite of truth that exists independently of the persons involved, it is a truth that is constituted anew by the patient and professional together, in each situation" (Gadow 1985: 38). Gadow sees the assistance of patients in defining their situation as an approach of caring (Gadow 1985: 38). According to her complex understanding of truth, it requires patients' participation in constituting it, and both, the patient as well as the nurse must be engaged. Therefore, she concludes the ideal of caring is an ideal of intersubjectivity, and "The alternative to caring as intersubjectivity is not simply reduction of the patient to an object, but reduction of the nurse to that level as well" (Gadow 1985: 38).

Gadow does not see a conflict between dignity and dependence. She thinks that dependence upon another for care of the body constitutes an indignity only when the person cared for becomes an object for the caregiver. Caring for the body, in her view, is important with regard to the phenomenon of *touch*. She outlines her thought as follows:

"Among all forms of human interactions, touch is the reminder that objectivity is not even skin deep. In touch, subjectivity exists at the surface of the body, and health professionals understand this perfectly. [...] Both, patient and professional tend to regard the patient's body as an object (and the professional's body as an instrument) in order that no bond be created or subjectivity invoked by touching. Technology provided a significant barrier in this respect. The stethoscope is safer than the ear to the chest, and the monitor, with remote viewer, removes the dangers of touching altogether. [...]" (Gadow 1985: 38).

I think the dichotomy between patient-oriented care and illness-oriented cure is based on a simplified understanding of medicine and nursing practices. Care and cure are often presented as if these concepts are irreconcilable realities and separate nursing and medicine. But, as medicine cannot be reduced to mere technological skills, nursing care is not free from handling technology. Many of the care practices are a matter of shared responsibilities since they are both ideally directed towards the realization of the same goal, that is the promotion of the patient's well-being. In palliative care physicians and nurses have to practice competent care including medical elements, such as pain alleviation. Especially in those fields where the collaboration of nurses and physicians are put into the center for achieving good patient-care, like hospice or palliative care, the existence of a dichotomy between care and cure can hardly be defended.

Caring as Charity and a Transformation of Compassion:
Back to Spiritual Roots

Jean Watson too, wants to contrast her idea of "care" with the medical model of "cure". She as the one who is holding the only "Caring" professorship in the United States (Colorado) has continuously working on her ideas about "caring" (1988, 1990, 1996, 2001). Her thoughts are based on the work by the human psychologists Abraham Maslow (1959) and Carl Rogers (1989) and hence, *needs* of the human being are regarded as central, and *trust* is seen as the basis for a caring relationship.

Building on the ideas of Gadow, Jean Watson opposed to Noddings, proposes a view of caring as the foundation of "nursing as a human science" (Watson 1985). Watson posits caring as human value that is characterized by "a will and a commitment to care, knowledge, caring actions, and consequences" (1985: 29). Like Gadow's understanding of care, such a view requires a commitment toward protecting human dignity on the part of the nurse (1985). Caring thus becomes a professional ideal.

For Watson, *spirituality* is a need as well as a power which is decisive for a humanistic orientated understanding of nursing. She describes her ideas about nursing by distinguishing the following components: (a) the charitable factors, (b) the transpersonal caring relationship, und (c) the caring occasion / caring moment (2001: 343–354). (a) The charitable factors are seen as the leading core for nursing. For her "care" means to meet someone with attention. (b) The transpersonal caring relationship implies that nursing takes over a moral responsibility of protecting patients' dignity and taking care of the spiritual dimension. To encourage the spiritual growth of the sick as well as those of the carers would be the aim of nursing. She remarks: "If we deal with human relational processes, the human wholeness of mind-body-spirit, and evolving human consciousness that is continuous with nature and the universe, we have to become part of the process" (Watson 1990: 20–21).

Jean Watson has mostly been criticized for being idealistic, for putting too much stress on psychology (Dunlop 1994). Philip Warelow remarks: "Some of her descriptions become lost because they tend to be far removed from the everyday practising nurse and are therefore banished to academic ivory towers" (Warelow 1996: 658). According to Sarah Fry, Watson's view of caring does not adequately support caring as a moral value and remains an ideal rather than an operationalized aspect of nursing judgements and actions (Fry 1992).

The Austrian nursing scientist, Silvia Käppeli (2004) has recently studied Watson's work and identifies her "feminine-caring-healing" approach as an attempt to rediscover an archetype of nursing that has been drowning in the course of the 20th century under what she sees as a male archetype of natural sciences (Käppeli 2004). Käppeli sees the traditional motivation of nursing in *compassion*. To have compassion for an ill and dying human being means to allow a relationship that includes trust and to know what suffering means for the cared-for (Käppeli 1988, 2004).

Care Ethics as a Mode of Defense against Dominant Models:
Challenging the Mainstream?

Unlike earlier writings that viewed ethics in nursing as primarily feminine etiquette (Aikens 1916, Gladwin 1937), the first books on ethics in nursing in the 1980s (Benjamin, Curtis 1986; Davis, Aroskar 1983; Jameton 1984; Muyskens 1982; Thompson, Thompsen 1985) view nursing ethics as a subset of contemporary medical ethics. Accordingly, they use the framework of bioethical principlism (Beauchamp, Childress 1983), theologically-based contract theory (Veatch 1981), liberal theories of justice like John Rawls' (1971), and Tristram Engelhardt's secular-based theory of human rights (1986). Sarah Fry (1989) realizes that this influence on the development of nursing ethics has been quite extensive. Discussion on ethical issues in nursing would be framed by deontological versus utilitarian theories and the weight of medical ethical principles rule nurse's decision-making processes in practice.

Fry criticizes that justice-based theories have almost exclusively been used in empirical studies of nursing ethics, and that medical ethical frameworks guide the majority of normative discussions of ethics in nursing. She explains that: "[…] autonomy and producing good were categories that the (nursing) researchers expected to find because autonomy and producing good are prominent features of medical ethics. What was assumed to be the case in medical ethics was assumed to be the case in nursing ethics, as well" (Fry 1992: 96). Fry criticizes that what appropriate is for the practice of medicine, would not necessarily be appropriate for the practice of nursing.

Moreover, with regard to language, she refers to Nel Noddings critique on a principle-based ethics that is represented through a language which only covers certain issues of concern while others get lost (1992). According to Noddings' "feminine understanding" of care, for Fry, care is foundational for nursing practice. She is concerned that an "ethics of caring" in nursing will not be able to survive in conditions of dangerous nursing shortages and monetary regulations unless nurses themselves insist that caring is central to their profession. This means that they must require sufficient time to develop care for themselves and their patients or clients so that it may be realized (Fry 1988).

Helga Kuhse (1995) vehemently argues against the idea of a "feminine ethics of care". In her article *Clinical Ethics and Nursing: 'Yes' to Caring, but 'no' to a Female Ethics of Care*, she harshly questions Watson's and Gadow's definitions of care for not being clear and she states her doubts about the feasibility of building an ethical theory on the concept of care alone but remarks: "Despite [...] inconsistencies and obscurities, [...] there is value in focusing on care as an important, but often neglected, component of ethics" (Kuhse 1995: 212). Kuhse understands caring as a disposition that helps to respond to the needs of others and contributes to a better patient care. She remarks: "[...] dispositional care is not only an appropriate part of nursing ethics, but of medical ethics as well" (Kuhse 1995: 213). Kuhse then explains that ethics is primarily about the justification of actions, and that "care" cannot be used as a reasoned argument (Kuhse 1995: 214). She is convinced:

"In the clinical context, such arguments will typically rely on certain universal principles, such as respect for autonomy or a health care professional's *prima facie* duty to act in the patient's best interests. To eschew all moral principles is to withdraw from moral discourse and to retreat into an essentially dumb world of one's own" (Kuhse 1995: 215).

For Kuhse, without principles there can be no ethical discourse and no justification, but "only particularities and unguided feelings" (1995: 216).

Theoretically disputable, on the whole, each of the presented concepts of care can be critically appreciated as a form of refusal to be co-opted by a rather abstract, principle-based kind of mainstream discourse. Still, on the whole, there seems to be a repetitive trap of falling into a polarized black-and-white discussion: struggling about "feminine" as well as "male" ascriptions and trying to balance as well as justify caring ideas against the principles like autonomy and justice.

Care Ethics from a Nursing Perspective in Germany

Although nursing has become an academic discipline within the last 20 years in Germany, its lobby is still weak, especially in comparison to the medical profession. Nurses are still struggling for more power and recognition, institutionally as well as academically.

In the 1970s and 1980s ethical issues of nurses were dominantly discussed by theologians and psychologists. Within the rise of ethics in health care, nursing ethics has become a sub-discipline of medical ethics. Nurses have hardly expressed their own position on ethical issues in health care within their academic discipline. Even though decision-making-processes like the governmental committees' work on Living Wills (see Introduction) will have a strong impact on nursing practice, their participation is missing.

Caring as a concept has mainly been discussed by theology and in medicine it is mostly seen as a sub-concept. Ideas of care are hardly received within the realm of German Nursing Science and caring as a practice has not been conceptualized yet.[23] Elisabeth Conradi (2001), a philosopher and political scientist, has developed a theoretical approach to a practice-ethic of care and highlighted its relevance to the practice of nursing (see Relational Analysis, chapter two). Also a few articles, published within the last decade, deal explicitly with caring and nursing. Wilfried Schnepp has developed his thoughts on the notion of the German word "Fürsorge" that is mostly used as the translation of "care". He discusses the notion of "Pflegekundige Sorge" that would rather capture nurses' capabilities (Schnepp 1996). The theologist Hans-Ulrich Dallmann (2003) dissociates from the ideas of caring as they have mostly been outlined in US-literature. Instead, he pleads for a theologically based nursing ethics that favors charity without ignoring the reality of conditions (Dallmann 2003: 15). The nursing scientist, Renate Stemmer argues against ideas about caring and nursing by referring to ideas about professionalism. She concludes in one sentence: "Despite these critical thoughts, it seems to me that the central point of the caring concept, namely that the care-giver has an interest in being basically attentive to the care-taker, has its essential meaning for nursing" (2003: 60).[24] Unfortunately, the "essential meaning" is not laid out.

Although there is an increasing number of German text books on nursing and ethics (Arndt 1996, Großklaus-Seidel 2002, Schwerdt 2002, Körtner 2004, Lay 2004) as well as some foundational theoretical studies (Bobbert 2002, Remmers 2000), literature about caring approaches in nursing is very scarce. In her textbook on nursing and ethics the nurse scientist Marianne Arndt (1996) has tried to integrate care ethics as "an ethic of women" by emphasizing the meaning of contextuality. Reinhard Lays' (2004) text book presents an enumeration of several understandings of an ethics of care and resumes an understanding of care as a "principle" (2004: 222). Caring as a practice of nursing is not discussed.

---

23 On how to integrate "Justice" and "Care" in the German discipline of *Medical Ethics* see Nikola Biller-Andorno (2001).
24 Translated by Helen Kohlen

Turning to those nursing authors who have considered caring, there is Marianne Rabe to mention. She has continuously been working on nursing ethics in its historical context. Rabe (2000) thinks that caring as an ethical orientation in nursing could probably be seen as the professional successor of the "old ideal of charity" (2000: 14). Elke Müller (2001) strictly refuses caring ideas due to a lack of theoretical knowledge (2001: 91). In her published dissertation *Pflegerische Verantwortung (Nursing Responsibility)*, Renate Tewes (2002) identified that most nurses understand caring as an essential part of nursing. She herself defines caring as a capability of nurses to attend to patients with frankness, dignity and respect (2002: 74).

In his work on scientific and ethical discourses from a perspective of a developing nursing science, Hartmut Remmers (2003) supports the idea of getting into a debate about models of care. He has continued encouraging a discussion about an ethics of care and situates it in the realm of virtue ethics. In an empirical study (2006) on caring from a patient's perspective who suffers from chronic wounds due to arterial obstructive disease, Perini et al. define care as a human interactive aspect of the nursing process (Perini et al. 2006: 350). In sum, the German scientific community in nursing has not yet critically examined ideas about an ethics of care.

2 Feminist and Nursing Studies in Care Ethics since 1990

Since this work has an interest in conflicts of medical and especially nursing practices that might currently be termed as ethical problems, foremost those theoretical approaches on care were selected, that seek to develop an understanding of caring as a practice as opposed to caring as a principle or an emotion. The literature study of the few theoretical frameworks that understand caring explicitly as a practice was lead by the following questions: Which theoretical frameworks (1) broach the issue of care within a broader political and social context, (2) provoke conflicts, including the ones experienced by nurses as a subject of discussion, and (3) raise questions about caring responsibilities? Moreover (4), do they imply a dimension that helps to understand and describe these conflicts beyond the bioethics style, and thus might provide a language and a framework for the analysis of the empirical data gathered in the field study of this work.

Joan Tronto (1994, 2006), a US-American political scientist, and Elisabeth Conradi (2001), a German philosopher and political scientist, meet most of the criteria pointed out in these questions. They have both situated care within its historical as well as socio-political context and claim its potential and need for change. Similarly, they argue to conceptualize caring as a practice. Most of the examples Tronto uses to illustrate conflicts of and within caring practices are taken from the field of nursing. Moreover, she considers nurses' professional competence from an ethical standpoint. Likewise, Conradi's work has nursing practice in mind. She sees non-verbal acts including touch as an integral part of caring practice and has outlined her understanding of nursing ethics as a part of care ethics. Tronto refers to the necessity of competence in the practice of care. The nursing scientist Patricia Benner has studied competencies in clinical nursing practice and her thoughts on care are of interest and her main discoveries are presented. Then, Margaret Urban Walker's work (1998, 2006) helps to understand care as a practice of responsibilities. For her, morality is not socially modular and something transcendent but a part of everyday social life. Walker's work is of interest within a social science perspective on morality and ethics and her framework helps to investigate how voices about caring issues get silenced. In addition, Walker has investigated into the field of clinical ethics consultation (see Historical Analysis, chapter three).

All of the identified theoretical frameworks turned out to be written by feminist ethicists.[25] Feminism as understood here, is not directly about equality and women but about power and its distribution in a specific cultural system like the health care system. Relations of power in any location, be it in the hospital or Hospital Ethics Committee, set the terms for who defines consequences; who has to question and who has to answer whom, and who gets excused from taking over (caring) responsibility of whom.

Caring as a Social Practice from a Political Science Perspective

Joan Tronto (1994) and Elisabeth Conradi (2001) see care first of all as a social practice that needs to be an issue of public and political concern. Tronto remarks:

"If we believe that there is good reason to take care seriously as a public value, then we will need to make three presumptions to provide such care. First, we need to presume that everyone is entitled to receive adequate care throughout life. Second, everyone is entitled to participate in relationships of care that give meaning to life. Third, everyone is entitled to participate in public process by which judgements about how society should ensure these first two premises" (Tronto 1994: 19).

Joan Tronto has continuously reminded her readers that care issues are far from being discussed as trivial and care work is absolutely necessary, it is currently devalued labor (Fisher, Tronto 1990, Tronto 1994, 2006). For her, it is not enough to assert any entitlement to care as if it were a good to be distributed. Instead, it needs to be seen as an activity of citizens in which they are constantly engaged. Tronto advocates, to acknowledge care practices is not that the state should become the provider of such services,

---

25 Patricia Benner does not declare herself and is usually not seen as a feminist, but in the introduction of her book with Judith Wrubel (1989) *The Primacy of Caring. Stress and Coping in Health and Illness,* she describes it as a feminist duty to make nursing work as a practice of care visible. Whether this work should be identified as a feminist duty might be related to the fact that most of these (invisible) care practices have been done by women. However, it is not outlaid by Benner, and not an issue that demands a more refined discussion here.

but that the state's role in supporting or hindering ongoing activities of care needs to become a central part of the public debate. Elisabeth Conradi has picked up Tronto's idea and understands care as a social practice that is shaped by certain conditions embedded in historical contexts. For Conradi, the conditions under which care is practiced are changeable and above all in need of reform.

Engaged Care and its Ethical Dimension in Joan Tronto's Work

Semantically, care is often associated with the notion of burden: to care means more than simply passing interest or fancy but the acceptance of some form of burden (Tronto 1994: 102–103). Joan Tronto found out that most of the definitions of caring presume that care is only an activity of individuals directed toward other individuals. "Not only does this exclude care for the self, but it also excludes the possibility that institutions or groups of individuals can care, or that people can care from a distance" (2006: 5). For Tronto, care needs to be understood as a universal aspect of human life that is done actively and responsibly. For Tronto, care applies not only to particular persons and things but as she suggests, to diverse practical forms including several services like nursing. Moreover, for Tronto, care should even be extended to politics. For her, moral theory is inextricable from political context, that is to say: Morality cannot be understood as separated from social roles and institutions. As such, following Tronto, care should be viewed as a political ideal in order to raise the status of both, care as a practice and those who do caring work. Consequently, she criticizes contemporary moral thinking for putting boundaries (a) between morality and politics, (b) between public and private life, and (c) between lived experience and the impartial moral point of view.

Defining Care as an Engaged Practice

Care conceptualized as a practice, in Tronto's view, is an alternative to conceiving care as a principle or as an emotion. It implies the involvement of thought as well as action. For Tronto, thought and action are interrelated and they are directed towards some end. This sort of engagement as she calls it, is not performed in an instrumental way and is different from the kind of engagement that characterizes a person who acts upon her temporary interests. Care means reaching out to something other than the self and is neither self-referring, nor self-absorbing. For developing a more precise account of care as a practice, Berenice Fisher and Joan Tronto offer the following definition:

"On the most general level, we suggest that caring be viewed as a species activity that includes everything that we do to maintain, continue, and repair our 'world' so that we can live in it as well as possible. That world includes our bodies, our selves, and our environment [...] all of which we seek to interweave in a complex, life-sustaining web" (Fisher, Tronto 1990: 18).

Tronto emphasizes that first, caring is not restricted to human interaction with others. But, the possibility that caring occurs for objects and for the environment is included. Second, it is not presumed that caring is dyadic or individualistic: "In assuming that care is dyadic, most contemporary authors dismiss from the outset the ways in which care can function socially and politically in a culture" (1994: 103).

Fisher and Tronto want to avoid a dyadic understanding since this might lead to a romantization of the mother and child relationship and the rest of society would be discharged from responsibility. Third, Fisher and Tronto insist that the activity of caring is largely defined culturally, and will therefore vary among different cultures. Fourth, in their sense, caring is not only seen as a single activity, but is also an ongoing process. In this regard, caring is not simply a discursive concern or a character trait but a concern of living that active humans are engaged in.

Four Dimensions of Care

Berenice Fisher and Joan Tronto have identified different dimensions of care. These dimensions are interconnected and can only be separated analytically: (1) caring about, (2) caring for, (3) care giving, *and* (4) care receiving. *Caring about* involves becoming aware and paying attention to the need for caring. Therefore it implies assuming oneself into the perspective of other individuals or groups. *Caring for* means to assume responsibility for the caring work that needs to be done. It also involves the ability to perceive one's power to actually act. *Care giving* is putting the actual care work into practice to meet the need. Most of the time the care-taker gets into direct contact with the care receiver. Here, nursing care as well as child-care are mostly used as examples (Fisher, Tronto 1990). Finally, Tronto describes *care receiving* as a fourth dimension: It is the response of those obtaining the attention and care. Otherwise, nobody would know whether caring needs have actually been met (Tronto 1994: 105–108). Tronto remarks that the fourth dimension of care "[…] can serve as an ideal to describe an integrated, well-accomplished, act of care. Disruptions in this process are useful to analyze" (1994: 109).

The question of conflicts arises and as Tronto remarks herself, care is not always a well integrated process but involves conflict. While ideally there is a smooth interconnection between these dimensions, in reality there are likely to be conflicts between as well as within each of these dimensions.

"Nurses may have their own ideas about patients' needs; indeed they may 'care about' patients' needs more than the attending physician. Their job, however, does not often include correcting the physician's judgement; it is the physician who 'takes care of' the patient, even if the care-giving nurse notices something that the doctor does not notice or consider significant. Often in bureaucracies those who determine how needs will be met are far away from the actual care-giving and care-receiving, and they may well not provide very good care as a result" (Tronto 1994: 109).

Another conflict often occurs when care-givers find that their needs to care for themselves come into conflict with their responsibility to care for others or that they are responsible to take care of a number of other patients or things whose needs collide with each other. Then the quality of care is put into question.

Ethical Elements of Care

In accordance with the identified dimensions of care, Tronto describes ethical elements of care: (1) attentiveness, (2) responsibility, (3) competence, and (4) responsiveness (1994: 127). The first ethical aspect of caring she calls attentiveness since care requires that a need is actually recognized and that this need should be cared about.

"If we are not attentive to the needs of others, then we cannot possibly address those needs. […] Yet the temptations to ignore others, to shut others out, and to focus our concerns solely upon ourselves, seem almost irresistible. Attentiveness, simply recognizing the needs of those around us, is a difficult task, and indeed, a moral achievement" (1994: 127).

The second dimension of care, i.e. *taking care of*, renders *responsibility* into a moral category. For Tronto, responsibility is a term that is embedded in a set of cultural practices, rather than in a set of formal rules or series of promises. It has different meanings depending upon one's perceived gender roles, and issues that arise out of class, family status, and culture Tronto remarks:

"Nevertheless, it is certainly possible for questions of responsibility to become political, in that they can become matters of public debate. [...] In arguing for the inclusion of care as a political and philosophical notion, I am suggesting that we are better served by focusing on a flexible notion of responsibility than we are by continuing to use obligation as the basis for understanding what people should do for each other" (Tronto 1994: 133).

The third dimension, *care giving*, stresses the importance of *competence* while care is actually given. Tronto argues that a central reason for including competence as an ethical element of care is to avoid the bad faith of those who would take care of a problem without being willing to do any actual care work.

"Intending to provide care, even accepting responsibility for it, but then failing to provide good care, means that in the end the need for care is not met. [...] But clearly, making certain that the caring work is done competently must be a moral aspect of care if the adequacy of the care given is to be a measure of the success of care. [...] sometimes care will be inadequate because the resources available to provide for care are inadequate" (Tronto 1994: 133).

Imagine, a nurse in an inadequately funded elderly home who is ordered to give care to demented people even though she does not know dementia care. Although she lacks competence, she does her best. The question then is, whether there is something wrong when condemning the nurse morally, since she hasn't produced the fault, but the reason is an inadequacy of resources. If the nurse is absolved from responsibility because she tries to do something beyond her competence, then good care becomes impossible. Those who have assigned the nurse can say that they have solved the problem without making sure that dementia care is actually occurring.[26] Tronto remarks: "Especially in large bureaucracies, this type of 'taking care of' the problem, with no concern about outcome or end result, seems pervasive" (1994: 134).

In any event as I see it, an important point about competence expressed here, is that competence requires professionals to engage in complicated and complex processes. The use of technical skills does not only demand being applied correctly, but at the same time adequately and coherently. Tronto remarks in her article *Does Managing Professionals Affect Professional Ethics? Competence, Autonomy, and Care*:

26　The exposition of this example is given by Tronto (1994: 133), but I have taken the freedom here to add on its complication, or better, the inherent conflict.

"Knowing when and how to broaden one's vision, without losing sight of the task ahead and without losing a sense of how to keep the task at hand as the central priority, seems also to be a part of genuine professional competence. To put the point in the language that I use in Moral Boundaries, professionally competent care-giving requires that one be attentive, responsible, and responsive at the same time that one is technically competent" (Tronto 2001: 193).

The fourth moral moment being implied in caring is responsiveness of the care-receiver to the care given. Tronto highlights that responsiveness suggests a different way to understand the needs of others rather than to put ourselves into their position (Tronto 2001: 136). To be in a situation of need means to be in a position of some vulnerability. Care is characteristically concerned with conditions of vulnerability and inequality, and thus, moral problems of responsiveness can arise. Since responding adequately requires attentiveness, moral elements of care are intertwined.

Care giving as the Central Part of Nursing Practice and Caring well

What can be resumed and might be considered about nursing care practice? As has been noticed, all of the moral dimensions of care that Tronto has identified are continuously involved in the process of care giving. Professional care workers like nurses will not separate attentiveness, responsibility, and responsiveness from competence as Tronto herself has pointed out.

Constant care giving is a central part of nurses' daily work while the other dimensions and elements of care are interwoven. In most domains of nursing like surgery or internal medicine, care giving is action-oriented and demands certain skills and handlings. This does not mean that the other dimensions and ethical elements play a subordinate role. On the contrary, then competence in the moment of care giving would be reduced to the correct application of techniques, and nursing would be no more than a job of daily chores.

The explication of one of the ethical elements of care induces the consideration of others. Finally, good care means that the fourth dimension of the caring process fits together into a whole. In like manner, to act properly within the framework of an ethics of care, the four moral elements of care are integrated into a whole. Of course, this is not easily done. Good intentions of a caring practice are not enough.

Care does not happen beyond conflict and power. Caring well requires looking at any caring process both in terms of the individual act of care necessary at a given moment as well as in terms of the entire caring process within specific contexts like institutional power-relationships. This implies the use of different perspectives to make sure that care is not being distorted by dynamics of those relationships of power and imposed or ignored needs. For Tronto, caring well

"[...] requires a deep and thoughtful knowledge of the situation, and all of the actors' situations, needs and competencies. To use the care ethic requires a knowledge of the context of the care process. Those who engage in a care process must make judgements: judgements about needs, conflicting needs, strategies for achieving ends, the responsiveness of care-receivers, and so forth. [...] Despite the fact that many writers about care concern themselves with relationships of care that are now considered personal or private, the kinds of judgements that I have described require an assessment of needs in a social and political, as well as a personal, context" (Tronto 1994: 137).

In Need for a Politics of Care

Tronto's point is that the ethics of care is incomplete without the politics of care. Unfortunately she does not explain what this would specifically demand and include. Generally, she remarks that a politics that considers care, recognizes and supports the caring labor that is crucial to the existence of society. It would shift the goals of social policy from securing an ideal of autonomy and promoting interests to taking care of vulnerable groups and meeting needs due to dependency. Even when citizens aren't self-sufficient they are valued. For Tronto, it is a myth thinking that we are always autonomous, and equal citizens. Assuming equality among people, leaves out and ignores certain dimensions of human existence:

"Throughout our lives, all of us go through varying degrees of dependence and independence, of autonomy and vulnerability. A political order that presumes only independence and autonomy as the nature of human life thereby misses a great deal of human experience, and must somehow hide this point elsewhere. For example, such an order must rigidly separate public and private life. But one reason to presume that we are all independent and autonomous is to avoid the difficult questions that arise when we recognize that not all humans are equal. Inequality gives rise to unequal relationships of authority, and to domination and subordination" (Tronto 1994: 134).

Tronto contrasts her position to the one she thinks, neo-liberals have: "Neo-liberals believe that encouraging the private pursuit of wealth, and limiting the public intrusion in the process, is the surest way to achieve collective happiness" (Tronto 2006: 3). Her converse position is: "Out of admirable personal conduct a public harm can arise. When unequal citizens only care privately, they deepen the vast inequalities and the exclusion of some from the real prospect of being full citizens" (Tronto 2006: 3). The ways in which the division of labor and existing social values allow some individuals to excuse themselves from basic caring responsibilities because they have other and more important work to perform, Tronto calls "privileged irresponsibility" (Tronto 2006: 3). She thinks, that as long as neo-liberals continue to insist that the separation of public and private life, accurately describes the limits of government's power, they provide an ideological justification for the deepening circles of unequal care (Tronto 2006: 3–4).

Eva Kittay shares Tronto's idea. Kittay has pointed out that an ethics of care belongs into the realm of politics and that care as well as justice need to be re-arranged (Kittay 2004). As long as care continues to shape the capacities of citizens differently, there can be no genuine equality among citizens (Kittay 1999).

The main critique on Tronto's work is that her concept of care would be too global. Tronto's definition of care can be seen as too broad by claiming that once you go beyond the person-to-person relationships you are doing something different than "care" (Held 1993, Ruddick 1989). While Elisabeth Conradi (2001) conceptualizes the practice of care in a similarly refined manner and refers explicitly to Tronto's work, she focuses on the person-to-person relationship.

Care as a Practice Ethics in Elisabeth Conradi's Work

Elisabeth Conradi (2001) understands care as a social practice that is shaped by certain conditions embedded in historical contexts. In her opinion, the conditions under which care is practiced are changeable and above all in need of reform. Conradi has tried to found what she calls a "practice ethics of care" and desists integrating care into traditional ethical concepts. Like Tronto, Conradi conceptualizes care neither as a principle nor as a virtue, but as a practice. She concedes that there is no precise translation of care into the German language and emphasizes that she does not understand care as an affective and instinctive matter.

Attentiveness, Interaction and Power Dynamics

Attentiveness, interaction and power dynamics are Conradi's key concepts in describing care as a practice. She characterizes care practices as interactions of being attentive and the receiving of attention. For her, care is sometimes even a matter of "giving attentiveness".[27] Her language of describing care as a practice is mostly related to Tronto's work. The similarities evolve especially in the translation from German to English.

On the whole, Conradi's work is based on different approaches: Care as a moral orientation of relatedness with reference to Carol Gilligan's work, and care as a practice of direct contact and engaged concern with main reference to Tronto. On this ground, she formulates nine theses about care (Conradi 2001: 44–58):

(1) Care is an interactive human practice: With the exception of self-care, it is shaped by at least two persons. (2) Usually the persons know each other, but also new contacts do evolve. In the process of the care-interaction a relationship between the involved persons grows. The making of contacts and the intensification of relations is understood as an activity. (3) Care encompasses the aspect of relatedness as well as care giving activities. (4) Care includes both, the actual care-giving as well as care receiving. Even to allow being cared for is seen as an activity. And, all participants, even though in different ways, are actively involved in the process.

(5) The asymmetry of care-interactions has a special meaning since the inherent dynamics of power need to be considered. Power differences do not automatically lead to humiliation, paternalism or subordination. Various forms of power differences within caring interactions can complement each other, and create tension. The question then is: How to perceive these power differences successfully in concrete situations and act accordingly?

(6) Although human beings within caring relationships show differences in their capabilities, competences and autonomy (*differently abled people*), attention needs to be developed independently of differences. The term attentiveness (Achtsamkeit) implies the meaning of attention by picking up its strong impetus as well as the meaning of offering care in such a way that people allow themselves to be cared for. (7) Attentiveness is not motivated

---

27 Asking Elisabeth Conradi by e-mail (2007), she agreed to the translation of the German term "Aufmerksamkeit" into the English one "attentiveness". She also remarked that "to give attentiveness" would present her thoughts, and declares "I speak of attentiveness rather than respect".

by reciprocity, but will always be a gift. And, even if reciprocity is an element in a caring relationship it will never be constitutive.

(8) Caring-interactions can be non-verbal, and in their broadest sense they are related to touch: Somebody feels touched by a situation or by the persons involved in the situation. Moreover, care has to do with physical touch: not only a face-to-face interaction, but likewise a body-to-body action can be a part of a caring process. Consequently, (9) feeling, thinking and acting are interwoven within care practices while the ongoing reflection combines all of these parts.

Criticism and Change within Practice

Conradi (2001) assumes that participants of care interactions perceive themselves as competent actors including being able to critically reflect a caring process. For Conradi, a critical evaluation cannot only exist beyond a concrete practice but also within the field of practice itself. That is to say, criticism and change do not need a direction from the outside but can happen within practice. In Conradi's view, criteria for a critical practice should be created within the frame of and in the procedure of concrete care-interactions. There are ways to justify moral judgement in specific situations without subordinating the particular to the general. Therefore, Conradi emphasizes the dynamic element that is embedded in a continuously critical contention of care interactions. Opportunities to tackle conventions critically can evolve in between subjects as well as inter-relational in the context of interactions and within institutional social conditions.

Nursing

Conradi (2003) herself has tried to apply her theoretical framework of an ethics of care to nursing. For Conradi, care is an essential part of nursing, and nursing ethics can be understood as a part of care ethics. She also remarks that at the same time nursing ethics might not be completely covered by care ethics. It is attentiveness that she thinks could be the starting point of developing an ethics of nursing. In her view, to conceptualize care in the profession of nursing could reveal its complexity, its moral dimension as well as the burden involved. This, Conradi insists, should no longer be put out of bounds. For her, putting caring practice off-limits implies its continuing devaluation and invisibility.

An important point about these considerations of care is to understand it as an interactive practice that enables the following: It allows the person cared for to flourish, which actually defines the purpose of care whether considered in the private realm or the public domain. The care relationship is not unidirectional towards the needy individual. It is not distorted by giving out care practices regardless of how it is received. The recipient of care is not passive, and care does not function in one way. Thus, caring as an interactive practice does not shape the recipient of care as a bundle of needs but puts the person into the foreground.

Nursing Practices of Care: Competence and Clinical Realizations

In their first studies, Patricia Benner and Judith Wrubel started out by viewing care as a "basic way of being in the world" (1989: 398). Apart from this rather abstract view, Benner points out that any study of nursing, including the study of understanding nursing care, should begin with practice (1989, 1994a, 1994b). In sum, her work has mainly been acknowledged for her empirical studies of intensive care nursing. Her main thoughts about nursing care practice and ethics will be outlined here. Based on a field study by Daniel Chambliss (1996), findings about how nurses understand care in the hospital setting will be presented. Mostly due to conditions given by the institution, the problems and conflicts nurses have to face when they want to practice care the way they think they should do it, are discussed in Relational Analysis, chapter two.

Expertise and Competence in Patient Care in Patricia Benner's Studies

Although it certainly does not capture Patricia Benner's phenomenological thoughts about care in depth, focusing on practice, it could be resumed that she has come to generally designate care as an attitude in form of a basic human concern and whenever care work is done, it is embedded in social practices that are framed by these concerns. Nursing belongs to those social fields where caring practices belong to the focuses of concern. Unfortunately, a technological and decontextualized understanding of health and illness leaves caring practices and social goods obscured and undermined (Benner, Wrubel 1989). Benner explains that as long as nurses would fulfill certain techniques and tasks without engaging in relationships one could not properly talk about *nursing practice* (Benner 1997). What did her numerous empirical studies show and how did she move to understand care as an ethical practice?

Studies presented in the book *The Primacy of Caring* make the importance of nurses' care practices visible (Benner, Wrubel 1989). Since nursing practice has mostly to do with patients who have to face a crisis, for Benner, "caring about" is an essentially required element on the part of nursing in order to cope successfully. The studies showed that nurses found out what was meaningful to the cared-for, which events were stressful and what resources and options were given to cope and could be accepted by the patient. Based on her study findings, in Benner's view, nursing practice is differentiated by various steps of care-expertise. To develop from a "novice" of nursing practice to an "expert" of nursing practice, *experience* is necessary. Her notion of "experience" entangles two sides, the first one implies a growth of knowing about how patients cope with health and illness; and the second one implies an increased knowledge about professional practice (Benner 1994b). Thus, she draws on a notion of *competence* that emphasizes the meaning of experience and its inherent growth of *implicit knowledge* (1994a, 1994b).

By investigating into the caring relationship between patient and nurse, in later studies, Benner and her colleagues could shed light on a competent nursing practice. It was asked what kind of competences nurses need to support patients in coping with their illness. Based on the findings, the authors point out that nursing competence also requires being capable to perform their duty in ever changing situations and to be confident as well as cautious about changing conditions (Benner, Tanner, Chesla 1996). Consequently, competence could be characterized by its flexibility of engaged care in complicated, complex, and changing processes.

In the course of her following empirical studies, Benner has come to see nursing as an ethical practice (1996, 1997, 2000). Following Benner, good nursing practice requires the following moral sources and skills: (1) relational skills in meeting the other in his or her particular life-manifestations of trust and openness of speech; (2) perceptiveness, for example, to recognize when a moral principle is at stake; (3) skilled knowing that allows for comportment and action in particular encounters in a timely manner; (4) moral deliberation and communication skills; (5) an understanding of the goals or ends of good nursing practice; (6) participation in community of practice that allows character development to actualize and to extend good nursing practice. All aspects of moral life are required for what she calls *phronetic nursing practice*.

Benner has mainly been criticized for putting too much emphasis on an ideal of nurses who embody a caring role and an ideal of a patient who allows to be cared for. Another critique that Patricia Benner as well as Judith Wrubel have been facing, is that they do not point out the inherent possible misuse of power within asymmetrical caring relationships and leave out institutional-structural conditions as being decisive for the quality of caring practices. For example, Joan Liaschenko remarks: "Making a voice for care but failing to attend to the realities of institutional life would be disastrous" (Liaschenko 1993b).

Hospital Care as Institutionalized Care

Caring in an institutional setting needs to be considered very carefully as it involves an ongoing interaction between two individuals of very different capacities and agency that carries the potential for abuse. Hospital routine is sometimes inconvenient or harmful to patients. Common complaints are sleep loss from frequent taking of vital signs and rising early in the morning for baths and medication. On the one hand, this arises from the efforts of nurses to allocate care to many patients. On the other hand, it results from short resources and inappropriate organizational culture of the hospital institution.

Based on his more than ten years field research in hospitals, sociologist Daniel Chambliss found out that the term "care" practically seems to include four meanings for nurses: "face to face working with patients, dealing with the patient as a whole person, the comparatively open-ended nature of the nurses' duties, and the personal commitment of the nurse to her work" (1996: 63).[28] A face-to-face encounter means fulfilling hands-on tasks like give baths, catheterize patients, turn patients in bed who cannot move themselves, and constantly watch patients with all five senses.

During the study, he observed, that nurses were constantly listening and talking to patients and relatives. While physicians visited floors to perform major procedures like inserting tubes into the chest, most of what was said

---

28 Chambliss remarks: "To a moderate degree, 'caring' describes what nurses actually do; to a great degree, it describes what nurses believe they *should* do" (1996: 63–64).

and physically done to patients was said and done by bedside nurses. Chambliss illustrates nurses' work in terms of spatial dimensions:

"The nurse works primarily in a contained space, on one floor or unit; if the patients are very sick, she stays in one or two rooms. She is geographically contained and sharply focused, on this room, this patient, perhaps even this small patch of skin where the veins are 'blown' and the intravenous line won't go in. She remains close to this small space, or on the same hallway, for a full shift, at least eight hours and in intensive care areas twelve hours; often she is there for two or even three shifts in a row. With the chronic shortage of nurses she frequently stays and works overtime. I have known a sizable number of nurses, in different hospitals, who worked double and triple shifts – up to twenty-four straight hours – on both floors and in ICUs. [...] So nurses have close contact with [...] patients over time, hour by hour if not minute by minute, for an extended period of time. [...] This close contact, over time, in a confined space, give nurses the sense that they know better than anyone else what is happening with their patients [...]" (1996: 64–65).

Although there were only a few nurses who actually delivered a continuity of care and only occasionally was one nurse responsible for the total care of a particular patient, nevertheless the geographical restriction to one area did cultivate nurses' knowledge of the condition of patients around them. Chambliss concludes: "To care for patients, then, first means that one works directly, spatially and temporally, with sick people" (1996: 65).

Moral Understandings and Responsibilities

Margaret Urban Walker's work *Moral Understandings* (1998) will be introduced shortly by the hypotheses she has developed in her book. Since Joan Liaschenko and Elisabeth Peter (2003) are nursing scientists who have fundamentally studied Walker's work, their thoughts are summarized. For resuming the ideas about feminist ethics and responsibility I will include a recent article by Walker (2006).

Moral Understandings in Margaret Urban Walker's Work

Walker calls her approach in feminist ethics a politically emancipatory one since it tries to be critical of the universalistic claim of contemporary moral philosophy. Her view of morality is alternative to the traditional understandings of morality: She thinks that theories of morality should not be confused with the human social phenomenon of morality.

In her book *Moral Understandings. A Feminist Study in Ethics* (1998), Walker develops an understanding of morality that consists in practices. She views moral knowledge as inseparable from social knowledge. Moral knowledge and moral practices are not extricable from other social ones. In particular ways of life they are entirely enmeshed with other social practices, moral identities, with social roles and positions. For Walker it is important to see that:

> "Morality [...] is always something people are actually doing together in their communities, societies, and ongoing relationships. It's not up to academic philosophers to discover it or make it up, even if it is, as I believe it is, a worthy task to try to understand it more deeply and to understand how it is open to criticism, refinement, and improvement" (2003: 175).

Central in Walker's view is the recognition that the human social world is a morally differentiated one. She rejects a moral point of view that excludes the moral context from individuality, relationships, history, needs, and context of the persons in specific situations. Her critique of the *"theoretical-juridical model"* is meant to clear space for an *"expressive-collaborative"* one she offers in her work. What are the main distinctions of these models?

Walker raises doubts about a certain view of moral theorizing and its allied conception of morality. The canonical way of moral theorizing, she calls the *theoretical-juridical model*, a template for what is usually seen as the genuine moral reflection. For Walker there could be a fund of purely moral knowledge only if morality completely transcended history and culture. In this taking of moral theory, moral ideas are transcended, idealized, and simplified by their abstraction from social practice. In Walker's view, this is unavoidable but leaves questions about how the social origin of ideas – created by philosophers who are socially situated themselves – shapes what their meanings can be, "whether novel applications we imagine for them can be achieved, and at what costs" (2001: 7). Against this model, Walker does not claim to create another moral theory (2003), but describes her methodological framework as "an exercise in transparency (that is) meant to test our thoughts about what we do and whom we take to be judges" (2003: 182). And: "Testing the moral authority of our practices means discovering how they actually go, what they actually mean, and what it is actually like to live them. [...] It means examining the power-bound social arrangements [...]" (2001: 10). For Walker, it is both: "A tool of normative philosophical critique as well as an actual social process that may be relatively inchoate and undirected or politically accentuated and mobilized" (2001: 9).[29]

In short, Walker sketches a culturally and socially situated, practice-based picture of morality that she outlines in four working hypotheses. The first hypothesis is to look at *morality as a set of practices* inextricably inter-twined with complex ways of living, in which people find the resources for understanding themselves. Moral concepts and judgements are an integral part of practices that "attempt to organize feelings, behavior, and judge-ments in ways that keep people's expectations in rough equilibrium" (2003: 176). The second hypothesis assumes that the practices to track are practices of responsibility: "People learn to understand each other [...] and to express their understandings through *practices of responsibility* in which they assign, accept, or deflect responsibilities for different things" (1998: 9). These prac-tices show who gets to do what to whom and who is supposed to do what for whom, and whose business anyone's welfare or behavior is (1998: 16, 2001: 6). Through such an arrangement of responsibilities "[...] morality 'itself' is *a disposition of powers* [...] requires many social powers. Powers to control, educate, and influence are required to cultivate and foster senses of respon-sibility" (2001: 6). Third, *morality is not socially modular*: Morality is neither a dimension of reality beyond or separate from life shared with others, nor a detachable and distinct set of understandings within it. Repetitively, Walker explains:

"Moral practices are not extricable from other social ones, and moral identities are enmeshed with social roles and positions. Moral understandings are effected through social arrangements, while all important social arrangements include moral practices as working parts. Just as there is no evidence of a distinct cognitive capacity dedicated to moral knowledge, there is also not any abstractable core of moral knowledge that completely transcends historically and culturally situated forms of society in which human beings learn how to live and judge" (2003: 176).

Walker emphasizes that moral concepts and judgements are an integral part, but only one part. Following from the third hypothesis, the final one is that the search for ideal, pure knowledge ignores differentiated moral-social worlds in which some people can demand accountability, assign responsi-bilities, and are themselves privileged to either accept or deflect responsibili-ties that come to them.[30] Typically there are *different responsibilities* assigned

---

29 In her book *Moral Understandings*, chapter three and nine give an in depth discussion.
30 For this situation Joan Tronto proposes the term "privileged irresponsibility" which re-fers to the ways in which the division of labor and existing social values allow some in-

to or withheld from different groups of people within the same society. The most obvious instance of this within societies is responsibility of able adults and older children for the young and incompetent. The practices of responsibility show what is valued and implies who is valued by whom (Walker 2001: 8). The belief that moral knowledge is pure hereby transcends the boundaries of a social world that is divided by race, class, ethnicity, religion, and gender. It rather shields moral theory makers from seeing moral knowledge as culturally situated (Walker 1998: 261). This search makes most of people's lives invisible, or render those lives unintelligible (Walker 1998: 10–11).

Walker thinks that the failure to situate particular universalistic moral views, especially when one believes they are indeed the correct moral views, "results in the curiosity, or the danger, of ethnocentric universalism" (Walker 2003: 177). She insists on the deep importance of seeing morality embedded in this way, as a real-time set of social practices that serves helping to keep safe the rich assortment of things that people most care about and that makes their forms of life habitable (Nelson 2000). For Walker, at "any moral-social order there must be trust that certain basic understandings are common and that the common understandings are the operative ones shaping shared life" (Walker 2003: 180). In Walker's view, morality thus becomes a collaborative enterprise, in which people reproduce and reshape the conditions in which they live with each other and understand each other and, of course, what Walker wants to be considered, is that not all of them have the same opportunities to settle or shift the conditions. Walker herself sees in the expressive-collaborative model a technique that aims both, to explicitly situate the projects of moral philosophy and to show where they are coming from by revealing the full complexity of the subject matter of ethics: "people's attempts – shared, but never fully agreed upon and always open to question – to sustain confidence that how they live is how to live" (2003: 182).

---

dividuals to excuse themselves from basic caring responsibilities because they have other and more important work to perform (Tronto 2005).

Perspectives of Nursing

Practices of responsibility are decisive while caring for the sick, injured, or handicapped people. This caring work is directed towards somebody who is in need in a particular situation and condition of dependency and vulnerability. These are the points, why, for example, Joan Liaschenko sees it as the moral work of nursing (1993a). Joan Liaschenko and Elisabeth Peter describe nurses as the "glue" of the health care system since they are continually being called on to negotiate and renegotiate their responsibilities for patients, families, other health care workers as well as the institution they are working in (2003: 261). Both authors have continued to apply Walker's understanding in the field of nursing. For them, Walker's analysis can shed light upon nurses' frequent sense of alienation with dominant bioethical theory, which falls within the theoretical-juridical model.

"Bioethical theory does not anchor nurses' identities, responsibilities, and the moral experiences of their work. At best, this alienation results in their concerns being discounted as 'ethical or moral problems' and redefined as merely practical problems. This dismissal or redefinition is a major way in which nurses' concerns 'get disappeared'. At worst, it leads to a moral self-doubt that calls into question the legitimacy of their concerns and their often highly astute moral understandings" (Liaschenko, Peter 2003: 261).

In her article, *Nursing and the Caring Metaphor: Gender and Political Influences on an Ethics of Care,* the nursing scientist, Esther Condon (1991) does also refer to Walker's ideas in her conclusion. She is convinced that the ethics of care must be informed with relevant knowledge. She claims that theories must be provided with knowledge grounded in the actual caring work and experiences of nurses, bringing theory and practice together in action.

"Actualizing an ethics of caring that avoids features of oppression and exploitation will also depend on the emergence of caring as a political philosophy capable of transforming institutions and the politics within which nursing is practiced, on removing bureaucratic barriers to caring practice, and on removing conditions that exploit nurses in the carer role" (Condon 1991: 18).

To resume the ideas about feminist ethics and responsibility, a more recent article (2006) by Walker, *The Curious Case of Care and Restorative Justice in the U.S. Context,* is helpful. She proposes to see care ethics in terms of three characteristics that point to facts of the human life-cycle.

As has been pointed out in my introduction, the first element of care refers to dependency as an inevitable part of it since everybody begins in fragile dependency. The second feature is the fact of vulnerability that implies that human beings have fragile bodies and feelings. The third one could be called the fact of interdependence that characterizes human social existence. "As we are dependent upon others for our very survival at the outset and at many times in our lives, we are dependent on many others throughout our lives for the necessities and amenities of a tolerable or a good life" (Walker 2006: 148). For Walker, these three facts encompass the primary information base of care ethics that is tapped by the question: "What do people need from each other to live well in the world?" (Walker 2006: 148).

Following the ideas of Joan Tronto and Elisabeth Conradi, but especially Margaret Urban Walker, I would like to point out: The work of nursing is constituted by practices of responsibility for those who are in need. Caring as practices of responsibil*ties* need to be shared by actors working on different levels of competencies: socio-political, institutional as well as relationship-based. What is of central interest in this work here, is the intermediate institutional level which can be seen as the micro-political one. As the work of the next chapter can contribute to: Care is not only practiced well when expertise and competencies of professional care-workers are given, but it also depends on enabling institutional conditions while those are connected to responsibilities of health care (macro) politics.

3 Concerns of Care, Conflicts and Nurses' Participation in Hospital Ethics Committees

The complexity of the health care system makes it difficult to locate the problems and concerns experienced by nurses. One way of sorting it out is as suggested above, to divide the places of action and decision-making into three levels. Described by an inside-out perspective there can be understood: First, the individual level; second, the institutional level; and third, the societal-political level. While conscientious objection is the resource to take a stand on the individual level, raising one's voice in public debates and going on strike marks taking a stand on the societal-political level. Besides joining the works council, participation in Hospital Ethics Committees offers a way to take a stand on the institutional level. One would expect that taking a stand on caring concerns and conflicts falls into the realm of nurses since they represent the biggest group to be involved in care practices. But, as this chapter will focus on: *Empirical studies* will reveal different findings.

Concerns of Care in Hospital Nursing Practice

Concerns of care in nursing practice are not uniquely a North American or German phenomena. Nurses in countries with distinctly different health care systems like England and Scotland, report similar shortcomings in their work environments and the quality of hospital care. A study in 2001 of more than 43,000 nurses practicing in more than 700 hospitals in five countries indicates that fundamental problems in the design of work are widespread in hospitals in Europe and North America (Aiken, Clarke, Sloane et al. 2001). Several studies have shown: while discontent among hospital nurses is high, a vast majority believes that the competence of and relation between nurses and physicians is satisfactory.

In North America and Germany, nurses reported spending time performing functions that did not call upon their professional training (delivering and retrieving food trays or transporting patients), while care practices requiring their skills and expertise (oral hygiene, skin care) were left undone (Aiken, Clarke, Sloane et al. 2001). Nevertheless, the problems of hospital nursing do not represent the entire profession. Tasks and settings vary widely.

Everyday Nursing Concerns and Invisibilities

The dominant concerns found in stories and narratives of everyday nursing practice are the ones of caring, responsiveness to the other, and responsibility (Benner, Tanner, Chesla 1996). Since responsiveness and responsibility can be described as elements of a caring practice (see Tronto in Relational Analysis, chapter two), it is the caring practice itself to be the issue of concern. What else has been found about nursing conflicts and concerns?

When the nurse scientist, and director of the Kennedy Institute Carol Taylor (1997) interviewed nurses to get to know their ethical concerns, she had to realize that most of the nurses felt hard-pressed to describe the nature of these everyday nursing concerns that had ethical significance. She states "[…] while some everyday nursing concerns are unique to nursing, most derive from tensions that involve the interdisciplinary team and raise broader issues about the human well-being that are best addressed by the institution or health care system at large" (1997: 69). In order to reveal their concerns, she then analyzed her collected case studies that lead nurses to request ethical consultation. She identified that nurses mostly struggle for (1) the respect for human dignity, (2) a commitment to holistic care, (3) a commitment to individualized care which is responsive to unique needs of the patient, and (4) the responsibility for a continuity of care and the scope of authority, and (5) identifying the limits of care-giving (Taylor 1997: 69–82). Taylor discusses that none of the concerns are unique to nursing although they may be experienced with greater immediacy and urgency by nurses as well as other care givers. She also observed that more nurses described their moral orientation as care-based rather than justice-based (Holly 1986).

The US-American nurse researcher, Joan Liaschenko (1993a) and the Canadian nurse researcher Patricia Rodney (1997)[31] have specifically in-

---

31   Pamela Bjorklund's article (2004) *Invisibility, Moral Knowledge and Nursing Work in the Writings of Joan Liaschenko and Patricia Rodney* gives an overview of various kinds of invisibilities. She differentiates between "unseen nursing", "unseen costs", "unseen harms", "unseen space", and "unseen knowledge".

vestigated into concerns of practicing nurses. In an ethnographic study of nurses practicing on two acute medical units, Rodney has explored the situational constraints that made it difficult for nurses to uphold their professional standards. Other research (Varcoe et al. 2004) supports her findings of experienced serious structural and interpersonal constraints, e.g. excessive workloads for nurses, the absence of interdisciplinary team rounds, conflicts between team members inside and outside nursing, and conflicts with patients and family members. Rodney gives examples of interviews with nurses where they described their attempt to provide nursing care for the elderly and critically ill patients as a race against the clock (Rodney 1997). She explains that the inability of nurses to arrange space to talk with patients, constrains their ability to truly focus and being attentive to the authentic needs of the patients and families. In a further study with her colleagues (Storch et al. 2002), in addition to a lack of time, another predominant theme was the nurses' concern about appropriate use of resources. They struggled with decisions made by others regarding the allocation of scarce resources. Some of the interviewed nurses in this study, described physicians as not willing to listen or to receive the nurses' point of view and were reluctant to accept that nurses have any independent moral responsibility when caring for patients (Storch et al. 2002). Megan-Jane Johnstone (1989) is convinced: "Anecdotal evidence abounds worldwide on how nurses are continually told by doctors that nursing practice is devoid of any sort of moral implication, and that it is nonsense for nurses assume that they have any independent moral responsibilities when caring for patients" (Johnstone 1989: 3). Yarling and McElmurry cite the case of an American physician who objected strongly to the suggestion that nurses have a moral duty, even though an attending physician has expressly ordered that not information be given out, to disclose information to terminally ill patients who request it (1986: 65–66).

Moreover, the study gave evidence that the organizational climate, including policy development had been problematic for nurses. Sometimes this was related to a lack of policy, sometimes to the presence of a binding policy, and more dominantly, to an ambiguous policy. For example, policies that were considered to be too binding, such as the resuscitation policies were related to patients whose best interest were overseen by following a code (Storch et al. 2002). Central to the concerns given voice by nurses that were interviewed in Liaschenko's study, was their sensitivity to patient need. They were aware of the

"[...] increased vulnerability to loss of [...] agency in the face of disease, illness. [...] Need was not seen solely in terms of a biomedical model of altered physiology but was conceived broadly to include those things which helped the individual to initiate or re-establish routines of lived experience and to cope with the settings in which they found themselves. [...] In this view, need was relative to the realities of the patient's day-to-day life" (Liaschenko 1993: 262).

The meeting of patients' and families' needs for emotional support, Liaschenko (1993a), Rodney (1997) and Varcoe et al. (2003) identified as being undervalued and overlooked in the work of nursing. "Because emotional work is a social transaction and not a product, it is invisible in a product-driven society. New nurses learn very quickly what the 'official' work is and what the unofficial work is. Emotional work is extra, frequently coming out of the personal time of nurses" (Liaschenko 2001: 2). The authors argue that economically driven changes imply that only certain processes are remunerated. Consequently, only certain, measurable aspects of care are accounted for and funded, while other tasks of nursing care are ignored. Hereby, different values underlie what gets accounted for and what is overlooked in an evaluation and a decision-making process that follows economic rules.[32] What also gets invisible in the work of nursing, is their dealing with social issues that have actually no place in the sphere of medicine and the mandate of the hospital like homelessness and poverty (Varcoe, Rodney 2001).

Liaschenko's identifies an unseen gendered space that nurses occupy in the larger bioethical landscape. She has shown how nurses can become actors who speak for others as "artificial persons", for instance, at the end of a person's life (1995b). Nurses bear witness to suffering at the end of life and try to alleviate that suffering when medical intervention stops. Liaschenko begins with the concerns of practising nurses as opposed to the bioethics issues of institutionalized medicine. For her, the concerns of nurses are often dismissed by the social order shaped by institutionalized medicine (Liaschenko 1993a,b).

In Germany, Rainer Wettreck has also used sight as a metaphor. In his grass-roots study he shows that nurses are stowaways in the hospital system, and that every-day nursing concerns are excluded by medically defined ethics, framed by those in a more powerful position (2001: 134).

---

32 Liaschenko remarks in this context: Since work is a key factor in how cultures differentially value and privilege different kinds of work, it would be central to how nurses identify, define and value themselves (Liaschenko 2001: 2).

Consequences of Distress and the Relational Organization

According to several research findings, there were significant personal costs associated with nurses' caring work and concerns: Fatigue, guilt, and personal risk as well as the experience of anger, frustration and feelings of powerlessness (Erlen 1993, Redman 1996, Rodney 1997). Nurses felt frustrated because they could not do what should be done with regard to "good care" and nurses felt powerless to affect their conditions of work (Rodney 1997). The constraints blocked nurses caring competencies and resulted in moral distress, that is knowing "[...] the right things to do, but institutional constraints make it nearly impossible to pursue the right course of action" (Jameton 1984: 6).[33]

Moral distress is said to be frequently experienced by nurses when they confront structural and interpersonal constraints in their workplaces. In addition, these constraints, the authors argue, are intensifying in today's era of health care reformation processes (Aiken, Clarke, Sloane 2000; Rodney, Varcoe 2001). Regardless of a certain conceptualization, the effects of moral distress are a serious concern. Webster and Baylis (2000) warn that unresolved moral distress can even lead to moral compromise and moral residue. Moral residue is what we carry with us when we knew how we should have acted but were unwilling and / or unable to do so (Mitchell 2001). Hence, the experience of moral residue cannot only encourage nurses to reflect on their practice, but the situation may also move toward denial, and trivialization (Webster, Baylis 2000: 224–226).

Lorraine Hardingham (2004) argues that nurses often find themselves in the position of compromising their moral integrity in order to maintain their self-survival in the hospital or other health care environment. The consequences are a fragmentation of care as well as fragmented decision-making that can have negative effects for patients and families and foster feelings of powerlessness and stress on the part of nurses (Varcoe, Rodney, McCormick 2003). But, of course, institutional constraints cannot be that easily be interpreted as a justification for nurses' behaviour. This can be no more than an explanation.

---

33 Moral distress is a concept that was first described in the nursing literature by the work of the American ethicist Andrew Jameton (1984). Since then it has been described as what individuals experience when they are unable to fulfill their moral intentions (Webster and Baylis 2000). Others define moral distress more broadly. Webster and Baylis state that moral distress may arise when a person fails to pursue what one believes to be the right course of action (2000: 218).

In a current study (2005), called *Power, Politics, and Practice: Towards a Better Moral Climate for Health Care Delivery*, Patricia Rodney has identified five themes as the main problems that are preventing safe nursing practice. Their participatory action research took place at the British Columbia Lower Mainland Emergency Department. In her findings, they mention first, the dangerous fact of "normalization":

"This means that serious congestion of patients in the ED, mismatches of patient acuity to available treatment / care, and overall lack of resources have started to become taken for granted. For instance, when asking hospital management for extra staff or to look for beds, nurses have told us (and we have seen) that the rebuttal is sometimes 'well, it was much worse the other day'. Nurses are sometimes asked to care for more than one ventilated patient plus other patients – a situation that would certainly not be considered 'normal' in a critical care unit. And patients are being held in the halls for so long now that some physicians are asking to start treatment in the hall or rapid treatment area without nursing coverage or assessment. This is in violation of safe emergency practice standards. Furthermore, it has become too much the norm that patients and their families will have to put up with far less than optimal care in our currently over-stretched provincial health care system" (Rodney 2005: 2).

Second, she points out of being "disconnected" which refers to the sense of nurses who feel that they are no longer connected to their colleagues, management, other departments in the hospital, or the community. Third, staff feel that they have no meaningful say in how the Emergency Department is run, but are rather expected to put up with the consequences. Overall, nurses told that they did not feel as persons and one participant of the research commented that she would feel as a "human doing" and not as a "human being". Rodney sees this as a form of "dehumanizing". Moreover, (fourth) "blaming", is one of the most dominant themes that cuts across every level of health care delivery. Rodney explains:

"While we have been engaged in our research, acute care and long term beds have been significantly cut in the region, and at the same time the regional population is growing. Yet the provincial health ministry has been blaming this health region for the problems in emergency departments [...]" (Rodney 2005: 3).

Fifth, as Rodney found out, it's "scarcity" as an overriding theme that affects all others.

In their book *Ethics on Call. A Medical Ethicist Shows How to Take Care of Life-and-Death Choices* (1992), Nancy Neverloff Dubler and David Nimmons remark with regard to the issue of "scarcity":

"[A] medical resource is classified as "scarce" whenever demand exceeds supply: when, for example, a hospital has one more patient in respiratory distress than it has available respirators, a respirator becomes a scarce resource. The medical assets in demand may be scarce because they are expensive, like intensive care beds in a hospital; they may simply be expensive, like highly technological devices called 'fluidized air beds'. Yet in each case, scarce resources confront caregivers with a lifeboat calculus where they must weigh which patient will benefit most from the resources available, and then choose. Often, that becomes a decision of who shall live and who shall die" (Neveloff Dubler, Nimmons 1992: 304).

A clear majority of US- and Canadian nurses reported that the numbers of patients assigned to them increased in the past year, which is troubling when considering the widely reported growth in patient acuity levels (Rodney 2005).

The reports from nurses in North America indicate that front-line nursing management positions have been eliminated in a number of hospitals. These findings imply that in addition to having responsibility for more patients, staff nurses might also have to take on more responsibilities for managing services and personnel at the unit level, and of course, which take time away from patient care (Aiken, Clarke, Sloane et al. 2001). One example given by Rodney (2005), is the insufficient acute and chronic bed capacity as a significant factor in overcrowding Canadian emergency departments. On the other hand, the study shows that strengths evolved. For example, the working relationships between nurses and physicians were identified as being strong and supportive (Rodney 2005). In a similar study, Rodney and Varcoe (2001) interviewed nurses who explained being in need of support by administration as well as by nursing leadership. Often, they described their nurse leaders as reluctant to raise nursing concerns. Some found help in reading ethics literature, by taking classes in ethics, and reference was made to the use of Hospital Ethics Committees. Nurses noted their reliance on nursing colleagues to deal with their problems in practice (Rodney, Varcoe 2001).

However, this "relational matrix" as Colleen Varcoe and her colleagues call it in a later publication (Varcoe, Doane, Pauly et al. 2004), will not be a guarantee for positive enactments of agency. Rodney gives the example of nurses who were put under pressure by colleagues to behave in ways that were obviously contrary to the good of patients, for example, the withholding of adequate pain management (Varcoe, Doane, Pauly et al. 2004). Hence, relationships in health care are important factors of health care outcomes for patients and the quality of work life experienced by health care providers.

Consequently, the quality of health care relationships needs to be a matter of concern as stated in the following quotation: "[...] we ought to be concerned about the effects of these relationships on care providers, especially with regard to their feelings of powerlessness and stress. In particular, what are the implications of health care relationships for the ability of nurses and others to provide 'good' care?" (Varcoe, Rodney, McCormick 2003: 959). In order to understand how the organizational context shapes relationships among patients, family members, and health care professionals, Varcoe and Rodney carried out a meta-analysis of their own ethnographic studies. They found out that

"[...] the notion of creating an organization to exert control over practice suggests that the relational matrix exists and functions, at least partially, to exert control over patients. The relational matrix can be seen to function, in part, as a mechanism to keep patients in line with the goals of the organization. Therefore, the relational organization can be seen as a network of connections among health care providers and between health care providers and patients – a network of connections within which power is enacted and agency is both constrained and facilitated" (Varcoe, Rodney, McCormick 2003: 963)

According to the authors, this understanding of the "relational organization", can help to appreciate the dynamic impact of the organizational context of practice. They resume that it can be seen as profoundly affected by structural changes in the health care context (Varcoe, Rodney, McCormick 2003: 964). What can these findings tell in sum?

I reason that nurses' issues of concern are systematic, that is to say: the problems arise in predictable settings and not randomly. The organization can make it very difficult for nurses to fulfill their ideals of good care. The ones who carry out caring work find it impossible to approach care as a coherent process. The fragmentation of care threatens the unity of the caring process. It is not something in the nature of *care giving* itself, but rather the low social status and the poor organization of care that can make nursing a difficult practice.

The meta-analysis shifted the understanding of moral distress (Varcoe, Rodney) since it revealed that it is not a linear process of cause (constraints) and effect (moral distress). Rather than focusing on individual action, Varcoe and Rodney came to see a network of individuals acting in relation to one another. Besides external constraints such as excessive workloads that got in the way of moral action, it was also how interconnected individuals acted in relation to each other. Nurses sometimes exercised coercive power over each other as well as over the patients and families they worked with.

They worked as operators helping to shape patients to the organization. "In defining patient problems in congruence with existing solutions [...] nurses functioned to reproduce, rather than challenge, the existing system and helped sustain existing hierarchies" (Varcoe, Rodney, McCormick 2003: 967). Nurses' moral distress here, can be no longer be seen as a consequence of their victimization by circumstances beyond nurses' control, but rather as distress created at least partially by their own participation in coercive practices and by distancing themselves from patients in accordance with dominant rules and practices. The authors conclude at this point:

"Although this [...] highlights individual nurses' culpability in using coercive power with patients and families to achieve organizational aims, it is the context of health care that shapes the relational organization and nurses' ability to enact moral agency. Thus, revising practice, rather than being the individual nurse's responsibility, will require a much larger and more collective effort" (Varcoe, Rodney, McCormick 2003: 967).

Since the concept of "scarcity" surfaced repeatedly during the analysis of the relational organization it served as a re-entry point into their data for analyzing the larger socio-political context. They asked, how "the ideology of scarcity" that was operating in the organizational context had its impact on shaping relationships (Varcoe, Rodney, McCormick 2003: 967).

For them, "the ideology of scarcity encompasses the taken-for-granted idea that specific services cannot be provided because needed resources are unavailable. Patients, nurses, physicians, and other care providers consistently spoke with acceptance about the inadequacies of time, money, and staffing" (Varcoe, Rodney, McCormick 2003: 965). The authors tell that they do not deny that there are real resource issues, but they want to point out that health care providers often take a passive stance toward resource allocation. When nurses talked constantly about the lack of time and resources required to fulfill their work, the authors observed that their talk was characterized by acceptance. Discourses of cost and cost containment were used to enable control over patients and of patient care practices. Cost containment was not only used to explain why desired services could not be provided, but over time patients and families learned that they should not even request what they wanted (Varcoe, Rodney, McCormick 2003: 965).

Varcoe and her colleagues found out, that these discourses of compliance were not only nurses' tools, but rather techniques that were essential to the maintenance of the organization:

"On a moment-by-moment basis, patients were deterred from making demands, for to do so would earn them sanctions for non-compliance, particularly for lack of compliance with the message that they should be frugal in their demands on health care providers and resources in the system" (Varcoe, Rodney, McCormick 2003: 966).

"Compliance" I think, could then be interpreted as an operation to afford nurses' control over practice and patient, and hereby becomes an efficient operational technique of the organization, respectively, the hospital. The question arises, whether health care providers always act in concert with these coercive dynamics and whether there are ways of resistance. The studies presented above reveal that there are practices of health care providers that can be resistant to imposed rules, changes and dominant ways of thinking. In these situations, individual nurses ignored rules and "the system" in order to practice care according to the needs of patients and families. The authors give the example of emergency nurses' practices of "bending the rules" to give patients pain medication to take home despite the lack of physicians' order (Varcoe, Rodney, McCormick 2003: 967). In sum, the researchers could see resistant practices as going against both: The prevailing ideologies and colleagues following them. According to these studies, the goals and rules of the institution can become the driving force for any kind of actions and procedures whereby nurses act as facilitators, negotiators, who are no longer dedicated to the well-being of patients, but to the system of management that implies a kind of *control over patients as cases*. What does it actually mean to 'know the case' in comparison to 'knowing the patient'?

Knowing the Case versus Knowing the Patient as a Person

Case histories and case records are part of a larger development of administrative technologies that can be called 'knowledge devices' are used by professions and in professional discourses as well as professional administrative practices. Procedures for writing them are manufactured in ways that records are collected according to standards so that the individual is put into categories and interpretative schemata as well as evolving caring practices. The facts are abstracted from the actual events that happened at a certain place in a certain time. Dorothy Smith remarks that they are "typically embedded in and integral to forms of organization where the immediate and day-to-day contact with the people to be processed is at the front line and involves subordinates, whereas decisions about those people are made by persons in designated positions of responsibility who lack such ongoing direct contact" (Smith 1990: 89). The structuring of the case story in this characteristic form, Smith explains, is articulated to an organization of power and position in which some have authority to contribute to the production of the textual realities and others do not. "Those who are the objects of case histories are normally distinctively deprived [...] those who have direct knowledge of the patient's life outside the hospital or of her daily routines in the hospital are least privileged to speak and be heard" (Smith 1990: 91).

Based on the analysis of their empirical research data, Joan Liaschenko and Anastasia Fisher (1999) differentiate between different types of knowledge that they call case, patient, and person. *Case knowledge* they consider as biomedical knowledge, that is the generalized knowledge of anatomy, physiology, disease process, and therapeutics (Liaschenko, Fisher 1999: 33–35). Liaschenko (1997) has claimed that case knowledge is "disembodied" knowledge. One could know, for example, all necessary facts about cardiac disease without perceiving that disease as being embodied in a particular individual. The disease is understood as a deviation from biological norm. Liaschenko and Fisher refer to research that was conducted in cardiovascular intensive care units and psychiatric emergency services. It showed that case knowledge is the one that nurses need to meet the primary goal of stabilizing, maintaining, and moving critically ill patients to another level of care. All of this knowledge proved to be biomedical knowledge that is the easiest knowledge to handle (Liaschenko, Fisher 1999: 34). Fisher and Liaschenko unfold the idea of case knowledge as followed:

"This case, or biomedical, knowledge is the primary knowledge of the contemporary health care system in that it legitimises the practice of medicine which, in turn, controls knowledge. It also legitimises that aspect of nursing work that is concerned with monitoring disease processes and therapeutic responses" (Liaschenko, Fisher 1999: 33).

And, according to Liaschenko and Fisher, this case knowledge is the standard, a standard against which the specific features of an individual care receiver are measured. The shift from case knowledge to patient knowledge is made when the care-giver encounters the actual body of the care-receiver. Hereby knowledge transcends case knowledge and grows to *patient knowledge:* The care of the patient at the bedside requires knowledge of how the disease is manifest in this particular patient. It includes any unique features of anatomy and physiology in this patient, and how this patient responds to care and treatments. For Fisher and Liaschenko patient knowledge also implies knowing how things get done for the individual within and between institutions as well as knowledge of other care providers who are involved (Liaschenko, Fisher 1999: 34–35). The authors remark:

"Part of the complexity of patient knowledge is due to the fact that its content is no longer limited to generalized case knowledge and the expectancies for action which it generates. Rather, it consists of the nurse's interaction with a particular body, the responses of which will be compared to generalized case knowledge" (1999: 36).

In contrast to case and patient knowledge, *person knowledge* is defined as knowledge of the individual within his or her personal biography (Brody 2002). It implies knowing something about what the specific history means to the individual.

Liaschenko's research showed that person knowledge was used when there was some conflict between courses of action desired by the individual and those desired by the therapeutic team (physician, physiotherapist, social worker etc.). Person knowledge is used by nurses "to defend their arguments for an alternative management of disease trajectories and to justify their actions when those actions support an individual's agency, even though this can conflict with established biomedical or institutional courses of action" (Liaschenko, Fisher 1999: 39). In other terms, this differentiation could be understood as a confusion of means and purpose. While the case knowledge assumes certain features that make up a certain profile of a person that fits the use of certain procedures, diagnostic techniques, and therapeutic possibilities, the person knowledge assumes an individual whose own biography and voice count to understand the case. Within the logic of the case knowledge, the individual can become a means to an end since you watch out for a profile that fits your available or prospective answers. Within the logic of the person knowledge, the individual is the purpose and transitional means and answers have to be found in the process of getting to know the individual by listening to his or her own voice and unique history. The person knowledge takes caring time and "understanding" becomes decisive while case knowledge saves time and understanding becomes unnecessary. The organization of care serves to separate the individual from the context in which interactions take place. To be taken away from that context means to become detached from the context of one's living. It becomes the organization's business. Individual histories can be rendered invisible or abstracted into a package of reports.

Nurses' Role and Participation in Hospital Ethics Committees

At first sight, it seems, if Hospital Ethics Committees demand multidisciplinary membership, nobody will question the membership and participation of nurses. But, as will be shown now, the literature analysis including research reports on this topic, as well as experiences laid out in expert interviews, a closer look is needed to understand the type of nurses' participation in these committees.

Participation denotes to be a part of and have a part in, for example a certain kind of program, process or political action. It means being involved in what is going on in one's field of work or interest. Participation implies acting together with other people within a certain environment or space, and hereby occupying a position in a process of institutional as well as social change. People have the chance or get the chance to play an active role, and: So do nurses with regard to Hospital Ethics Committees?

Nurses' Role in Hospital Ethics Committees

From their start, Hospital Ethics Committees have recognized the importance of including individuals from different backgrounds as members. The legitimacy of the nurse's role and the potential contribution of professional nurses as members of these committees has been acknowledged by diverse authors (Aroskar 1984; Fost, Cranford 1985; Fowler 1986; Judicial Council of the American Medical Association 1985; President's Commission 1983; Youngner et al. 1983). Nursing as well as medical literature gives attention to the benefits of including nurses in ethics deliberations. Nurses are supposed to add further dimensions to the decision-making process because they are usually in close proximity to their patients and spend more time at the bedside than any other member of the health care team. Thus, nurses have a special understanding of benefits as well as burdens that medical treatments have on patients.

The overall given argument for nurses' participation in Hospital Ethics Committees is that nurses have direct *contact with patients*. Since nurses are the ones who would spend more time with the patient and families than any other professional group they would have a incomparable knowledge about the patient. To be mostly involved in patient care situations can bring a perspective to the committee as nobody else can (Murphy 1989). They are seen to have expert knowledge in the communication process and as members of an ethics committee, they are expected to be the ones who primarily collect data and express questions, viewpoints and perceptions of patients and families. Hence, their membership can provide a formal channel to communicate their observations. Moreover, nurses are often the ones of the health care team who are familiar with all the players of the conflict. "The nurse can alert the committee to various factors that may confuse the situation and conceal the major ethical issues. For instance, fear of legal consequences rather than ethical principles may threaten to guide decision making" (Murphy 1989: 555). The handling of communication can be seen as the most important competence since it has been commonly acknowledged that clarifying the facts and *fostering communication* comprises 80 percent of an ethics committee's work (Youngner et al. 1983).

For the description of nurses' role in Hospital Ethics Committees, the term patient *advocacy*[34] is mostly emphasized. For example, Patricia Murphy remarks in her article *The Role of the Nurse on Hospital Ethics Committees*:

"Nurse members who act as patient advocates must articulate and defend the autonomy rights and interests of the patient. To be an advocate involves informing and supporting. Nurse advocacy occurs when the committee promotes effective communication; learns the reactions of patient, family and staff; increases patients' knowledge about their illness; and encourages more participation by nurses in the informed consent procedures" (Murphy 1989: 554).

Judith Erlen thinks, that a "basic understanding of ethical principles and moral reasoning is essential for the nurse in order to identify, articulate and resolve dilemmas in clinical practice and strengthen their role as a patient advocate" (1993: 70). Amy Haddad critically comments on the emphasis on patient advocacy:

---

34 The term "advocacy" has its roots in the legal system. Before the advocacy model was supported, nurses believed that their primary obligation was to obey physicians and maintain order within hospitals. This military sense of nursing identity originated in the context of the Crimean war, when Florence Nightingale brought order and improved conditions in hospitals (Bernal 1992: 18). Apart from a discussion on nurses' role in Hospital Ethics Committees, the advocacy model gained wide acceptance among US-American nursing scholars in the 1980s. The ideal of advocacy has been viewed as important in furthering nursing's endeavours on behalf of those actually or potentially in need of nursing care (Curtin 1979, Gadow 1980, Kohnke 1980). The specific features of patient advocacy have continued to be debated, For example, Ellen Bernal (1992) questions the debate on nursing and advocacy since it would idealise the image of autonomy by impoverishing a view of social relationships, illness, suffering, and the obligations of the professional to the patient. Pamela Grace also raises doubts about advocacy as a practice ideal. She stresses the need for a wider concept that shifts the attention to nurses' professional duty and responsibility (2001).

"You know, that is interesting, because this is a term that I have never been cautious about. And I think it is just the side of being paternalistic, although, of course, it is, the use of the term it's meant all out of good! What I mean, what nurses bring, and what is important, is not just representing the patient's view which I think advocacy sees it, I am going to speak for them. What I mean is, what is it like in the life of a patient, that are people that are more removed from that [...] don't have any idea [...]. That kind of insider witnessing to people who are suffering, to the struggles that they are having. That is important" (Haddad 2005, see Appendix 1.2.2).

Haddad prefers the use of the term *witnessing* since advocacy for her "[...] always sounds legal to be and paternalistic. It moves very quickly speaking for the patient without any input from the patient and the family" (Haddad 2005, see Appendix 1.2.2). She emphasizes the following importance of nurses' role:

"I think they have to speak about their experience at the bedside, and be able to articulate about that. I have the experiences over the years, that nurses are very quick to claim: we are running around for 24 hours [...] So, yes, what is important about being with the patient for 24 hours a day and being closest to the patient, is what you see, and hear and learn and that needs to be brought to the table. Because nobody else has that information. Not to say, I am important, you know, I am there [...] use what you know from there and bring it to the table. This is something they will hear, especially, of patients whose families are not present. Because they (the families) bring that perspective too" (Haddad 2005, see Appendix 1.2.2).

Nurses' Membership, Voice and Participation in Hospital Ethics Committees

"Membership indicates who can speak, whose opinions are counted, and whose discounted. Membership may determine even which issues are seen as legitimate ethical concerns and which are not. [...] So, to say that a hospital has an ethics committee tells us very little unless we know as well: who serves on the committee and under what authority" (Bosk, Frader 1998: 16).

What are the experiences of nurses with regard to membership, participation, and bringing in their voice? In 1991, a study on *Physicians' attitudes toward Hospital Ethics Committees* found out that merely 69 percent believed that nurses should be members in clinical committees and only 59 percent thought that they should have access (Finkenbine, Gramelspacher 1991), and when the number of Hospital Ethics Committees had drastically risen, the US-American nurse ethicists Barba Edwards and Amy Haddad (1988) remarked that the specific and unique ethical concerns of nurses had also not been adequately addressed by these multidisciplinary committees. Their issues were not framed as ethical issues and therefore excluded. The nurse ethicist Dianne Bartels who co-chaired a Hospital Ethics Committee in Minnesota in the 1980s is convinced: "I do not think hospital nurses have trouble speaking up, they just need a place to show up. [...] you need a place to convene, and then, once you are there, people don't have trouble [...] representing their issues." She also thinks that the co-chair model equalizes power, expands interaction on the committees and increases the comfort of nurses to be able to speak up. Moreover nurses need to "learn the language"[35] (Bartels 2004, see Appendix 1.2.2) to be able to discuss the issues. What does it mean to "*learn the language*"?

As early as 1986, Cheryl Holly revealed in her dissertation on *staff nurses' participation in ethical decision making*, that nurses are forced to function at conventional levels in bureaucratic organization of the hospital. It was seen as a failure when they couldn't define concerns related to their practice in terms of rights and justice. Nurses who attempted to operate from a base of caring and responsibility were relegated to a conventional role. Betty Sichel examined procedures, deliberations, goals, and functions of Institutional Ethics Committees, and realized that "a rights and just model is not appropriate, even though and ICE must often consider legal dimensions or precedents"(1992: 119).

Published in 1990, a descriptive study on *Participation and Perception of Nurse Members in the Hospital Ethics Committee* gives a detailed overview that reveals change compared to the findings before (Oddi, Cassidy 1990). The study was conducted in two phases. In the first phase they determined the number of acute care hospitals in a Midwestern state that have Hospital Ethics Committees and to obtain the names of the nurses who serve as members of these committees. In the second phase, they contacted individual nurses to assess the extent of their formal involvement in ethical decision making as well as their perception of the role of the ethics committee within their institutions. Of the 148 responses from hospitals, 45 percent said having an ethics committee. All hospitals reported that nurses serve on those committees. The average number of nurses was said to be two. The identified nurses were invited to participate in the study by anonymously completing

---

35   Interestingly enough, some minutes later in the interview, she was looking out for words to describe a concern given to her by a nurse. She interrupted herself, saying: "Sorry, I am afraid I am losing my nursing language" (Bartels 2004, see Appendix 1.2.2).

a brief questionnaire about their perceptions "[...] of how the ethics committee is involved with selected aspects of practice" (Oddi, Cassidy 1990: 309). Members were predominantly female, hold a master's degree, and served in administrative or management roles. The mean age was 42 years with a range of 25 to 65 years. The majority reported that they were either appointed or had volunteered to serve on an ethics committee. They also indicated that they served on the committee from one to seven years, with an average tenure of two years. Academic preparation, continuing education, and self-directed learning were declared to be the main ways in which nurse members learn about ethics. Completion of an ethics course at either the graduate or the undergraduate level was reported by more than half of the respondents. Most of them indicated that they had attended continuing education programs, conferences, or workshops on ethics. All respondents indicated that they contribute comments and ideas to the discussion of the committee. Only a few indicated that they sometimes contribute, over 40 percent stated that they usually contribute and nearly half said that they always contribute to the discussion. Only 1.4 percent indicated that their input was seldom sought by the committee (Oddi, Cassidi 1990).

The nurses interviewed in a pilot study by Storch and Griener (1992) were generally positive about the perceived potential of a Hospital Ethics Committee, but only a few nurses were actually aware of the presence of the ethics committees. For example, at one hospital, 20 nurses out of a total of 361 respondents were not aware of any ethics education being offered by the hospital. The study found that differences in ease of access to Hospital Ethics Committees by health care professionals were particularly pronounced between physicians and nurses. Physicians seemed to have greater access to the ethics committees, and were perceived to have more support from these committees. In contrast, nurses did not perceive themselves as having direct access to the hospital ethics committee for consultation. They considered that access would be through their supervisor. Even though these "gatekeepers" posed no significant barrier, a few nurses interviewed, stated that they would be too intimidated to go to the Hospital Ethics Committee. Non-nurses commented about the nurses' access to the ethics committee frequently and more openly than most nurses. Social workers were the ones who explicitly declared that nurses had limited access to the Hospital Ethics Committees, "[...] because a nurse's desire for a consultation could be 'squashed' easily by a physician" and others stated that nurses' concerns are not well addressed (Storch, Griener 1992: 23).

Another reason for nurses having difficulties in gaining access to ethics consultation or even ethics discussions is the status of ward or unit. Although the physicians interviewed in the study by Storch and Griener thought that good interdisciplinary consultation was practiced on their units, and although many head nurses agreed with them, the staff nurses on those units did not share this perception. Some of them thought that their voices were not heard, and that they felt silenced in ward consultations. Some nurses find it reassuring that an ethics committee exists, but they also said that day-to-day ethical concerns are being ignored (Storch, Griener 1992).

Cornelia Fleming found out: "In institutions with established Hospital Ethics Committees, nurses are routinely included as members; however, the number of nurses able to participate at this level is small and not proportionally representative of nurses in clinical practice" (Fleming 1997: 7). Here, a problem evolves: The locus of the conflict is at the bedside of the patient, nevertheless, not bed-side nurses as actors of caring practices participate in Hospital Ethics Committees, but nursing managers. While nurses in management may bring a broader view, the special perspective of staff nurses may be lost if they are not adequately represented. This is actually a contradiction to the given role of nurses pointed out above, since nursing managers do not know patients by direct contact, do not witness their particular situation, and thus, cannot communicate the caring knowledge staff nurses usually have.

Although an occupation may have an adequate numerical representation, there could be differential participation in terms of communication exchange as the study by Charlotte McDaniel (1998) reveals: In her qualitative research she examined nurses' communication exchange frequency as members in four sample Hospital Ethics Committees. Nurses represented the same or more membership numbers as physicians in proportion and the frequency of nurses' communication exchange was comparatively modest in proportion. The nurses had one of the smallest proportions of communication exchanges. Although most of the nurse-members contributed communication exchanges to a topic, there were also nurses who did not participate at all. Nevertheless, nurses rated their participation effectiveness quite high. This rating is one of the highest among the occupations represented on these committees and contrasts with suggestions that nurses feel unqualified and unprepared. Although nurses were moderately communicative on the committees, McDaniel suggests: "[...] nurses are engaged, active, and selectively participating in the committee deliberations. Nurses appear to be comfortable with a less overtly active, yet representative numerical membership on the committees" (McDaniel 1998: 50). These findings suggests that concern for adequate representation and participation of nurses may be due less to the actual numbers and due more to the interaction on the committee. Further exploration of the content of nurses' communication showed that they participate most in the discussions regarding patient care. Communication revealed less activity with regard to policy formation and education. McDaniel argues that nurses representing the single largest group of healthcare personnel need to be involved in the policies and decisions that surround and affect their administrative and clinical practice (McDaniel 1998: 48). McDaniel reflects that several explanations relevant to nurses may be explored to further understand the outcome. She observed that every group member is undoubtedly influenced by the committee composition and dynamics, including, for instance, the chairperson, the size, or the topic of the discussion (McDaniel 1998: 50).

A research project by Sarah-Jane Dodd, Bruce Jansson, Katherine Brown-Saltzman and their colleagues, published in 2004, investigated the extent to which nurses engage with regard to two kinds of behaviour: First, "ethical activism"[36] in trying to make hospitals more receptive to nurses' participation in ethics deliberations. Second, "ethical assertiveness"[37] where they participate in ethics deliberations even when not formally invited. The researchers contend that these two kinds of involvement are vitally important if nurses want to expand their ethical roles. The results indicated that nurses are more likely to employ ethical assertiveness and ethical activism in settings that are already receptive to nursing participation. The results also showed that ethical assertiveness and ethical activism are closely related to each other, that is to say, nurses who scored highly on ethical activism also scored highly on ethical assertiveness. From the lack of receptivity to nurses' participation in ethics deliberations in some of the hospital settings in the sample, the researchers conclude, that far more attention should be devoted to ethics training. Moreover, they think:

---

36 Ethical activism they defined as "actions directed toward reforming institutional policies and procedures, as well as attitudes of physicians and other medical staff, to create favourable climate for (nurses') participation in ethical deliberations" (Dodd, Jansson, Brown-Saltzman et al. 2004: 17).

37 Ethical assertiveness is defined as "actions to enter or facilitate ethics deliberations in which nurses have not been included, whether through personal initiative, coaching patients, advocating patients' wishes to others, or ethical case finding" (Dodd, Jansson, Brown-Saltzman et al. 2004: 17).

"[Nurses] need to try to change the hospital environment so that it promotes, rather than discourages, their participation. Even when not formally invited, (they) need to engage in ethical assertiveness when they advocate for patients, coach patients, act as ethical case finders, initiate ethics deliberations, and not withdraw from deliberations when not specifically asked to participate" (Dodd, Jansson, Brown-Saltzman et al. 2004: 26).

For several obstacles related to questions of class, gender, colour, level of education, religion or other social markers that do mostly shape rather stable power-structures in a hierarchical institution like the hospital, and hereby orders who should ask and answer what to whom, who should take care of what, and has the authority to change something (Dodd, Jansson, Brown-Saltzman et al. 2004: 26).

Changing processes implies effects on others, other individuals and groups as pointed out here, the encouragement of nurses' participation. If nurses think this might be a good idea, this does not mean that everybody else welcomes more nursing activity. Especially not those who might occupy a position that is threatened (Haddad 2005, see Appendix 1.2.2). From the perspective of the nursing hierarchy (staff nurses, ward leaders, management, directory), each group occupies its special space, and it is usually the task of nursing management who should have influence on the shape of hospital environment, but, as the studies by Patricia Rodney and Colleen Varcoe (2001) have shown staff nurses do not see that they are supported by them. What are the questions that can be raised at this point?

The findings of the studies I summed up, raise the question, whether ethics committees support existing structures and power relationships in the hospital rather than provide a means for more collegial decision-making and increased interdisciplinary discussion of conflicts and dilemmas. The comments from physicians, nurses and administrators give credence to the view that Hospital Ethics Committees merely support the existing power structures. A second puzzling question is why the nurses might know so little about ethics committees. Storch and Griener ask whether this goes back to a lack of knowledge that is induced by medical politics or whether it could be understood as a strategy of nursing administration maternalism that keeps staff nurses and head nurses removed from such information, or whether it might be simply a problem in communication within the hospital (Storch, Griener 1992: 25). When I asked the nurse ethicist and director of the Center for Health Policy and Ethics in Omaha, whether Hospital Ethics Committees have in some way changed power relationships, she remarks: "Yes, I mean, just the whole question who can ask for an ethics consultation changes the power structure. And if you open it up to anybody who wants to ask for assistance, then you change who is in charge" (Haddad 2005, see Appendix 1.2.2).

In sum, the US-American studies on participation of nurses in Hospital Ethics Committees between 1980 and 1994 (Edwards, Haddard 1988; Oddi, Cassidy 1990, McDaniel 1998) show that nurses participate most in discussions that pertain to patient care review or to particular clinical situations. Nurses are less active in discussions regarding policy formation and even less active in discussions of topics pertaining to education. Judith Erlen concludes: "If nurses are to [...] fulfill their professional responsibilities [...], then resources for nurses have to be developed and made available within each health care agency" (1993: 71). She reminds that the standards issued by the Joint Commission on Accreditation of Healthcare Organizations in 1992 had required that structures be in place within institutions to enable nurses to participate in ethical deliberations (Erlen 1993). This standard is also included in the *Standards of Clinical Nursing Practice* developed by the *American Nurses Association* in 1991. But, having structures build up that nurses can have an easy access does not necessary mean that their voices are heard, and their language of defining an issue of (caring) concern is understood. The nurse ethicist and nursing manager Hans de Ruyter who has more than ten years of committee experience in two different hospitals has gained a rather critical perspective and explains:

"Nurses' issues get addressed if they present them the way that the people, the physicians and the kind of the leadership see it. So, you have to present it in a certain way, and if you go outside of that model, [...] so, if you bring up an issue that they do not classify as being an ethical issue, you don't get listened to. But people and nurses, I think, we are very adaptable, so there is always nurses that will learn the language and you get listened to [...] But then, you cannot truly bring up the issues that you think are ethical issues because it's very much I think with ethical issues which issues are classified as ethical issues and which ones aren't. And, I think that the nurses who do that and I can't talk about [...] their mind, but for me, the quandary is. Do I want to be a part of the leadership and then I have to adapt, or do I speak what I think should be spoken, and that automatically makes me an outsider" (De Ruyter 2004, see Appendix 1.2.2).

Nursing Ethics Committees

There are nursing professionals who have established Nursing Ethics Committees (NECs) as entities separate from the multi-professional Hospital Ethics Committees. These committees are structures within the healthcare organization created specifically to assist nurses in resolving dilemmas. They are comprised of nurses who represent the different positions of nurses within the organization, such as nurse managers, nurse educators and staff nurses and are supposed to assist nurses to identify, clarify and articulate the issues in their practice (Erlen 1993, Fleming 1997).

A forerunner of the idea could actually be dated back to the time when the institutionalization of Hospital Ethics Committees after the Quinlan decision first subsided. At that time, in many hospitals, still some rather small and unknown groups began to meet regularly to discuss clinical problems they were facing with their colleagues (see Historical Analysis, chapter three). Ruth Purtilo told in the interview in 2005 that to those unknown groups belonged a group of nurses at the Massachusetts General Hospital (MGH) in Boston in the mid 1970s. She explains:

"A group of nurses came to me telling 'We need an informal committee', [...] what they needed, was a room and time to talk about daily conflicts and dilemmas in clinical practice. We established an informal forum to discuss nursing ethical issues. The goal was to get this forum more or less institutionalized. One effect of the forum was the reduction of moral distress" (Purtilo 2005, see Appendix 1.1).

Purtilo recounts that nurses could deliberate about dilemmas, conflicts or distress among peers that they encounter in clinical practice and identify strategies for nursing action. Issues that were purely nursing concerns could appropriately be discussed in such a forum that allows familiarity (see Appendix 1.1).

One of the first official Nursing Ethics Committee was established in a Catholic hospital in Omaha, Nebrasca in 1984. The vice president of patient care, Barba[38] Edwards, took the initiative to establish a Nursing Ethics Committee at the hospital, because she couldn't get the Multidisciplinary Ethics Committee moving (Haddad 2005, see Appendix 1.2.2). Amy Haddad, professor and director of the Center of Health Policy and Ethics at Creighton University in Omaha, and at that time doctoral student of nursing, became a consultant. Interviewing her, she explains:

---

38 Her name actually is "Barba" and not Barbara.

"[...] when once the Nursing Ethics Committee was started and had a full day orientation to what ethics was, how decision would be made, how to structure it [...] we had representatives from all the nursing areas in the hospital. This is before the hospital had governance structures, so there wasn't anything else in place [...] we got the people who were most interested to do it. So, we probably met for six months, people on board for [...] physicians to establish the institutional ethics committee. So, I had to work as a consultant to that committee [...] both committees (!) the Nursing committee and the committee for the whole institution" (Haddad 2005, see Appendix 1.2.2).

Haddad and other authors have proposed Nursing Ethics Committees as a resource group since they would focus on education (Edwards, Haddad 1988; Erlen 1997; Zink, Titus 1994). The forum is also described as a way to empower nurses so that they can more fully participate in multidisciplinary ethical discussions and prepare nurses to become "effectively involved in Hospital Ethics Committees" (Zink, Titus, 1994: 70).

At first glance and from the perspectives given above, establishing NECs seems, to be an adequate way to address issues of conflict and care, but also critical considerations are expressed. Erlen argues that nurses who discuss issues only with other nurses might be limited in their focus. Perspectives given by other healthcare workers could challenge the analysis of the conflict and broaden the enquiry. "Although all nurses do not hold the same exact philosophy of nursing, there is a greater likelihood that there will be less divergence of perspectives and fewer alternatives presented when an ethics committee is comprised almost entirely of nurses" (Erlen 1997: 59). Nursing Ethics Committees might encourage division rather then collaboration with other disciplines (Fleming 1997: 8). Besides, clinical ethics expert, Mary Faith Marshall points out in an interview, since "nurses can be their best enemies" and a "democratic process" should be learnt, change in practices of local multidisciplinary committees need to be supported by everyone (Marshall 2005, see Appendix 1.1).

A closer look reveals that the question could be raised whether the functions of Nursing Ethics Committees are often the responsibility of other committees within the healthcare organizations. While some nursing concerns are unique to nursing, most raise broader questions about human well-being that might be better addressed by the institution and the healthcare system at large (Taylor 1997: 69). Moreover, a restricted discussion of these concerns to Nursing Ethics Committees may end up in their becoming trivialized or even marginalized. The separate committee might communicate the image to the institution that these concerns are of lesser importance than those addressed by an interdisciplinary committee. And there remains the question to ask: What happens if the committee actually serves to make nurses grow stronger in articulating their thoughts and put their issues of concern on the agenda? Haddad tells about her piece of history:

"It created problems over the years because they stood up, collectively, you know, so you got now five people on the unit, and they are not only five people, they are five experienced people because usually people that volunteer for this had been there a while. And now we are going through years of running the committee, and learning a language and all that. Then you got five people who were saying, we are not going to put up with this. They started to present problems [and there came a new director]. She was unhappy with how they [the nurses] reacted to [...]. I mean, they had learnt to ask questions. They had learnt to say that they would not agree on policies: We are not following it. Why are not following it in this case, so what is happening? They had learnt to use tools of good arguments. [...] They had been taught to tell why [...] you cannot go up to somebody and say you are wrong, you have to have good arguments, and be able to say, here are my concerns and this is why [...] and they had been taught to do that, and they had learnt to link arms in how to do that, because nobody wants to be the one going forward" (Haddad 2005, see Appendix 1.2.2).

Participation as an Idea of Democratizing Hospital Ethics Committees?

As the study results revealed, 'participation is not just participation'. There can be multiple possible ways of participation, as long as they haven't been taken on, nobody has had participated in this sense.

The Australian political scientist, John Dryzek (2000) favours what he calls a discursive instead of a deliberative form of democracy. Whereas "deliberative" can be a personal decision process and not necessarily a collective process at all. He stresses that the deliberative form does not involve communication, whereas a discursive process, in contrast, is social and has intersubjective aspects, and necessarily involves communication. He adds:

"[...] deliberation has connotations of calm, reasoned, argument. This is unnecessarily constraining and renders the model vulnerable to those who point out that this sort of gentlemanly discussion is not a good paradigm for democracy. A discursive process connotes something much more expansive in the kinds of communication it allows, *including unruly and contentious communication from the margins*" (Dryzek 2000: vi; emphasis added).

Moreover, Dryzek points out that the term 'discourse' draws attention to two traditions of political theory "that, though attaching different connotations to the term, are central when it comes to making sense of deliberation" (Dryzek 2000: vi). The school of thought that follows Michel Foucault, Dryzek explains, compares a discourse to a prison because it conditions the way people think. According to a different school of thought that is influenced by Jürgen Habermas, discourse has the opposite meaning since a "pure freedom in the ability to raise and challenge arguments" is presumed (Dryzek 2000: vi).

Following Dryzek, fostering participation can take place along the following three dimensions. The first is franchise: Expansion of the number of people capable of participating effectively in collective decision. The second dimension refers to scope which means: bringing more issues and areas under democratic control. And the third one is authenticity of the control which signifies to be real rather than symbolic and involves the effective participation of autonomous and competent actors (2000: 29, 86). Specifying his notion of democracy, democratisation takes place if, (1) the presence of the hitherto scarcely represented group increases among the actors who are actively involved in the decision making process, (2) the implication of inequality and power relations being bound to traditions is seen as a problem to be expounded in the decision making process, and (3) the decision making process meets the criteria of unconventionality and reflection as well as modification (Dyzek 2000: 86–87).

Bringing these bottom lines forward to questions with regard to the participation concerning nurses, the first dimension of franchise could be: Do nurses who have hitherto scarcely been represented participate in Hospital Ethics Committees, and are they actively involved in the working processes and collective decisions? With regard to the dimension of scope, questions could be: Is the implication of power relations within institutional and clinical practice seen as a problem to be expounded in the decision making process? Are nursing issues and areas brought under democratic control? Does the institutional culture and structure support the democratic framework? More to ask with reference to authenticity is: Does the clinical ethics decision making process meet these criteria? Is nurses' participation real rather than symbolic?

Taking these ideas to analyze the research findings about nurses' participation in Hospital Ethics Committees that I outlined before, one can conclude that their participation does not necessarily mean that their issues are raised and their voices are heard. Power relationships being bound to a traditional institutional hierarchy in hospitals is not seen as a problem to be expounded. Finally, it appears to be that nurses' participation is a type of participation that is symbolic rather than real. For the process of taking participation in a sense of a discursive process seriously, it would be important to consider in what kind of institutional culture the Hospital Ethics Committees are built up, and see what kind of organizational structure is needed to meet the criteria that I pointed out above. Moreover, it is decisive to take care of the direction problems are raised and discussed, the language that is used and the "prison" that might be built up.

4 Summary

By tracing back ideas about caring and an ethics of care I could identify circles of polarizations. When Carol Gilligan initiated a care versus justice debate, care was going to be interpreted as a feminine approach and her emphasis on context for processes of decision-making was taken up and set against a principle-based approach. The debate continued to be primarily being driven by women who tried to raise attention to those dimensions of *care* that they felt were neglected or even ignored in dominant theoretical debates and too much detached from their own experiences: The meaning of relations, context and dependency. There are no transitions of thought in the development of the care-ethics debate in the 1980s, but circles of polarizations like care versus justice and touch versus technology. What changed were the areas of application like in the field of nursing.

While Patricia Benner has specifically studied nursing as a *practice*, Joan Tronto – and later in Germany, Elisabeth Conradi – have studied caring as a social practice that needs to be an issue of public and political concern. Tronto describes care practices by distinguishing between four different dimensions that carry ethical elements of care. For her, the first dimension, *caring about* involves the ethical element of *attentiveness* since care requires that a need is actually recognized and that this need demands to be cared about. The second dimension of care, that is *to take care of* cannot be separated from *responsibility* as Tronto explains. She sees responsibility embedded in a set of cultural practices rather than in a set of formal rules. The third dimension, *care giving* stresses the importance of *competence*. Finally, with regard to the fourth dimension, *care receiving*, Tronto highlights the meaning of *responsiveness*. She points out that care would be characteristically concerned with conditions of vulnerability and inequality, and hence, problems of responsiveness can arise.

Margaret Urban Walker understands morality as a human social phenomenon that consists in practices of responsibility. Within the same society, she explains, there are typically different responsibilities assigned to or withheld from different groups of people. The practices of responsibility show what is valued and what is devalued. With regard to caring practices of responsibility, Tronto has pointed out her concern about "privileged irresponsibility" since there would be ways in which the division of labor and existing social values allow some individuals to excuse themselves from basic caring responsibilities.

The analysis of nursing science studies on hospital care revealed that the organizational context of caring practices are profoundly affected by structural changes in the health care system. The organization can make it very difficult for nurses to fulfill competent care that meets their moral expectations. The research has repeatedly shown that a fragmentation of care threatens the unity of the caring process and "knowing the patient" well. Nursing hospital care is marked by a low status, a poor organization and a *marginalization* of care.

US-American studies on nurses' participation in Hospital Ethics Committees have revealed that they are included as members of these multidisciplinary forums. Yet, their number is rather small and not proportionally representative of nurses in clinical practice. At the same time, their *active* involvement is limited. While they are mostly involved in discussions that pertain to patient care review or specific clinical situations, their nursing care concerns are not adequately addressed. On the contrary, their issues were not framed as ethical issues and therefore excluded. The necessity of "learning the (ethics) language" as one nursing professor in an expert interview remarks, then implies that nurses' issues might get transformed into ethically acceptable problems that do not hit the point of caring conflicts.

Questions that are of interest for the empirical work that is presented next are, whether and how caring issues and conflicts are addressed, and in which way this is linked to the participation of nurses.

Practical Arena Analysis
Practices in Hospital Ethics Committees
in Germany

1 Introduction of the Field Research

> "Practice has a logic which is not that of the logician.
> This has to be acknowledged in order to avoid asking of it more logic
> than it can give, thereby condemning oneself either to wring
> incoherencies out of it or to thrust a forced coherence upon it."
> *Pierre Bourdieu, The Logic of Practice*

The field research took place in Hospital Ethics Committees of three different hospitals located in the North and in the South of Germany. Including the survey to find comparable committees in size and time of establishment and the validating of the interviews after the participant observation, the empirical study required a length of three years. Fortunately, the problems that were met by the researcher could either be practically solved or lived through in an adequate way so that the long time of empirical work was neither distorted, jeopardized, nor invalidated. The fact that I have a nursing background helped to get entree into the clinical field of the unknown hospitals. Background knowledge of clinical work helped not being seen as a disembodied recorder of someone else's actions, and could certainly contribute to trust-building. Nevertheless, the field study fully demanded the effort to keep the strength of participant observation and to reduce its inherent weaknesses as much as possible (see State of the Art, chapter three).

Method

Selection of Committees, Entrance into the Field and Cooperation

The field research was prepared by a survey to identify the hospitals that had started to build up an ethics committee nearly at the same time to allow comparison. This was worked out by the attendance of conferences on Hospital Ethics Committees (University of Essen 2002, Academy of Tutzing in Munich 2003) and by contacting (by e-mail or telephone) actors in the field who would turn out to be door-openers for the research.

Out of five clinical ethics forums that had started in 2003, access for the field research was given by three door-openers of the following hospitals: (A) Protestant hospital (525 beds), (B) Catholic hospital (400 beds) and (C)

Municipal non-university hospital, now privatized (570 beds). The Privatized[39] and the Lutheran hospital are both located in the North of Germany, and the Catholic one is located in the South. While the privatized and the Catholic ones are Hospital Ethics Committees according to the classical US-model *(Klinisches Ethikkomitee)*, the Lutheran hospital has established an open forum without standing membership, called "Round Table Dialogue-Ethics". Besides being open for everybody's participation in the hospital, its tasks are also structured along the US-model. Therefore, despite its difference in structure, the Lutheran forum is also called a Hospital Ethics Committee in this work.

All three hospitals were rendered anonymous by fictive names. The Lutheran one is called Hospital *Ast*, the Catholic one, Hospital *Bach* and the municipal / privatized one, Hospital *Clön*. Moreover, the names of the field subjects were made up by naming all the ones of Hospital Ast with an "A" in the beginning, like chairperson Dr. Arras; all field subjects of Hospital Bach begin with "B", like ambulatory care nurse Mrs. Busch, and the one of Hospital Clön with a "C", like the Lutheran minister, Mrs. Carr (see Appendix 2.1).

The preparation for the field research involved the arrangement of meetings with key persons that would allow the entrance into the research setting. Therefore, contact was established by e-mailing and telephoning as well as meetings with the door-openers, the chairperson(s) of the committees and leadership persons to get formal permission for the research. I explained that I was doing a dissertation on Hospital Ethics Committees and that the field study would involve participant observation and interviews. They all were curious about the research and arranged formal consent from the hospital directory. Only the head of the Lutheran hospital showed some reservations. He expressed being afraid that the presence of the researcher could influence the activity of the committee participants in a way that was no longer "controllable". Nevertheless, he gave his permission.

Before entering the actual research field of Hospital Ethics Committees, a separate meeting with the chairperson(s) took place in each hospital. Details of the research process were explained and questions of confidentiality were cleared. On the premise that real names of persons, places, and so forth would be substituted by pseudonyms or not mentioned at all, the chairpersons gave some oral background information about the start of the committees as well as access to documents like standing orders and the

---

39 This hospital has been privatized since 2005.

minutes of committee meetings that could give hints to working procedures and rules.

At the first meeting (entering) of each forum that I attended (see Appendix 2), I introduced myself, described the research by handing an outline to the members, assured them of confidentiality, and asked them to introduce themselves so I would know what profession and discipline they were representing. I indicated that if at any time they wished me to leave, I would. As part of the negotiated entrée, I offered to return after the study was finished and share what I had learned from all the ethics committees visits. All three ethics forums were positive about my role as a participant observer, and asked some rather formal questions.

Trust-building has been decisive from the beginning of the field research in order to make sure that the planned sequenced participant observations of the Hospital Ethics Committees' meetings could take place over two years (2004–2006). Access being allowed in the field, is one thing, but approval and trust of field subjects is quite another. Cooperation cannot be ordered by leadership, but is rather earned step by step and a continuous process. During the whole field research a continuous communicative contact by e-mail writing and telephoning was kept to the committee chairpersons. The strategy of "passionate detachment" (Haraway 1988: 585) – defined in this study as developing relationships with committee participants and reflecting upon these formal trustful contacts – was successful. Questions with regard to additional information and explanations that would help to clarify confusions and give a contextual understanding of the collected data had always been immediately answered by the chairpersons.

Finally, leaving the field required a careful way of getting out. Trust relations that have been set up needed to be respected and participants in the research needed to be reassured that they will not be abused, misrepresented or exposed to potential harm by the researcher's use of the data. Contacts are retained for the purposes of subsequent clarification or in the event of subsequent research.

Gathering Data in the Field, Preparation and Interpretation

The oral information that was given in the *first meetings* with leadership persons of the committees and directorship of the hospitals as well as the information gathered by the study of the standing orders and minutes brought out three case stories of the selected Hospital Ethics Committees. In addition to the data, the organizational structures of each Hospital Ethics Committee could be summed up.

The *first visit* (entering) in the committee of Hospital Ast, Bach and Clön served to get accepted as a participant observer and get to know the structural data like membership, time and space. In the following, the first up to third or fourth participant observations were more and more *focused* and connected to the research questions. Then, the final *selective* observations (fourth or fifth to sixth) were turned to central aspects that could validate or discard preliminary findings.

My role in the meetings was primarily to listen and observe. Sometimes I asked questions that would help me to understand abbreviations or actions related to how things are handled specifically in the hospitals. I did not comment on the ethical issues during the meetings, although several times people asked for my advice. The committees seemed more and more to accept my presence and the fact that I was taking notes.

I observed a total of twenty-three meetings with an average number of six observations in each committee. The hand-written observations during the meeting were typewritten afterwards and when questions evolved they were clarified by questioning the committee chair persons. Before the selected observations took place, the data of four focused participant observations in each committee was summed up and structured along communalities and differences of committee tasks and functions as well as along the evolving topics of committee discussions.

Following the steps of qualitative content analysis (see State of the Art, chapter three), the first part of the data analysis was to reduce the data by abstracting it in such a way that the substantial content was kept. The process of thickening the observational data led to a corpus for explication. Then, field notes and interviews were used to supplement the process of preliminary interpretation. A thematic analysis was done for each participant observation respectively for each transcript corpus. Hypotheses were developed and I discovered where the data was rather weak and where the observations needed to be concentrated on in the future.

As the research moved along, and the familiarity with the field increased, the original research question was both broadened and re-evaluated. It seemed of most relevance to inquire how the brought up "ethical problems" were defined, how issues of conflict and concern were denoted and connoted as well as what kind of matters of care practices evolved and disappeared within and beyond case discussions. Other changes were also apparent at the time, influencing my focus. One was nurses' and physicians' framing of concerns, their way of participation in debates, their silences, their absence and sudden way of leaving the committee.

The observations and the preliminary results of the first analysis were discussed within a group of graduated university colleagues and supervisors. Then, the research questions were refined and the next attended committee meetings were characterized by an observation of selected aspects. Gradually relationships between themes were identified and descriptions of the findings developed. A level of saturation was reached after six to seven participant observations in each hospital. All the typed up participant observations were put into tables and translated into the English language (see Appendix 2.4). Like any translation does, this detailed work with words and phrases implied a first step of interpretation. The table shows who speaks, what is told and how the people act during committee meetings (including disturbances). It also contains an explication of what is said by the committee participants and in one column reference signs are given.

In addition to the participant observations, the twenty-eight informant interviews (see Appendix 2.2) provided essential context-relevant as well as clarifying information that was needed to explicate and validate the observational data for interpretation. Moreover, subjective meanings for the participants could be identified and shed a different light on the relevance of some observations for the evolving research findings. Not only committee members and irregular committee participants, but also people of influence outside the committee served as informants (see Appendix 2.2). The influence of people outside the committee (non-participants) was mainly revealed during committee discussions. The informants had to be carefully questioned by the researcher in order to piece together the particular facts of the events from which the researcher himself was absent. Most of the informant interviews were done when the fieldwork had been completed, and the data had been summarized into its final substantial corpus.

Furthermore, gathering necessary information made it necessary a few times to spend some time talking to other personnel of the hospital, like hospital administrators and nursing staff of the intensive care unit (ICU). The manifold ways of data collection, information gathering and steps of analysis while gradually structuring the material along themes, give confidence in the validity of the inferences that I have drawn.

The Case Stories

In all three hospitals, the documents created during the design phase of the ethics forums, like standing orders or preambles as well as the minutes of their first meetings refer mainly to membership and functions which are taken over from the US-American model. Looking from the outside of the ethics committees in hospital Ast, Bach and Clön, they do all look quite alike. The interviews with directorship, leadership persons as well as people from outside the hospital could reveal different contexts and motivations for each committee establishment. Each history influenced the type of the forum, leadership, membership and participation.

Background of Committee Establishment

The motivation to establish a Hospital Ethics Committee is related either to problems that can be traced back to the past, or by facing current re-organizations of the hospital. The history of the ethics forum in the Lutheran hospital (Ast) goes back to an "[...] ethics project undertaken by Dr. Amburg (a professor of Ethics and Public Health), a couple of years ago" (All 2005, see Appendix 2.2.1). As Dr. Amburg explains, this ethics project involved interviews with physicians and nurses, and revealed that a lack of communication between professional groups was having negative effects on patient care. Therefore, the head of the hospital, the minister, Mr. All, had strongly been pushing the committee idea for fostering a "culture of dialogue" in the hospital. "Nevertheless, significant problems of communication are very old and persistent in this hospital" Mr. Amburg points out in the interview (Amburg 2005, see Appendix 2.2.1).

In the *Catholic hospital* (Bach) the building of an ethics committee is strongly connected with the prior existence of a palliative care unit. After attending a conference on Hospital Ethics Committees, the senior palliative care physician, Dr. Boha, took the initiative to talk to people in the hospital about the idea of an ethics committee. He said that talking to people over a long period of time gave him the feeling that questions about *end-of-life issues* were growing. Among those issues raised by nursing staff, questions on when and how to "end therapy" were dominating as Mr. Buth, the head nurse of the intensive care unit informs (Buth 2004, see Appendix 2.2.2). Dr. Boha thought that especially for those questions being raised by people working in intensive care and the associated elderly home, an ethics committee could be helpful. His idea was supported by the head of the hospital, some other physicians, the nursing manager, and: "The head physician of palliative care and anaesthesia had been very strong to foster the establishment of the committee" (Boha 2004, see Appendix 2.2.2).

In the *Municipal hospital* that was recently privatized (Clön), the initiative to establish an ethics committee was born within the dynamics of its preceding working group, called "quality management and pastoral care". The female minister, Mrs. Carr, had played a decisive role of "geting people again around a table to discuss what really needs to be discussed" as Mr. Commer, the committee chairperson explains (Commer 2005, see Appendix 2.2.3). A male senior physician (internist, Dr. Ceisch) and a male nurse (nurse, quality management, Mr. Commer) who had been in the preceding working group are the ones who asked people in the hospital to become members of the ethics committee. Most of the ones who were asked, agreed (Commer 2005, see Appendix 2.2.3).

To summarize, in the Lutheran hospital it is the "old" problem of communication, and the Catholic one is connected to past issues of end-of-life care. In the Municipal hospital, the committee work is the result of the hospital privatization. It developed out of a working group during the reforming process, called "quality management and pastoral care".

Organizational Structures and Participation

In the following I will present the organizational structure of each hospital in the field research and look at participation with a focus on nurses. A table at the end of this part gives an overview of the structural data with regard to membership, leadership and frequency of meetings.

The meetings of the open forum "Dialogue – Ethic Round Table" in the Lutheran hospital (Ast) are officially open to anybody working in the hospital. There is no close membership and anybody who has an interest in joining the committee meetings can do so. Usually about twelve to sixteen people attend and show more or less activity in the discussions. The meetings do usually take place in the afternoon and usually last two hours. The participation is included into the regular working time or can be counted as overtime if someone participates in her or his free time.

With regard to leadership, the head of the Lutheran hospital (minister, Mr. All) had asked another male theologist (Dr. Arras) and a lawyer (Mrs. Amt) to chair the committee. While Dr. Arras does not work at the hospital, but works at a center for health care ethics, Mrs. Amt works at the hospital. The leadership persons organize quarterly meetings that take place in conference rooms of different buildings.

The observations revealed that they actually do not have "round tables" but sit at long tables and the two chairpersons do always sit at the top. Consequently, the participants do not look at each other, but their eyes are constantly focused on the chairpersons. When questions are asked their reactions are focused on the chairpersons while the moves by the others remain rather unseen. Therefore, committee members who feel neither addressed nor really involved in the conversations take the time to do other things, like communicating with the messages on their mobile phone: Calling and being called have been constant interruptions during the meetings. The open forum model and the name "Dialogue Ethics Round Table" turned out not to be real, but rather symbolic since the table is neither a "round" one to foster a communication of dialogue, nor is it open to everybody in the same way since some persons are actively invited.

Although everybody is invited to participate in the committee meetings, people are once in a while explicitly invited to participate. The number of nurses who do participate varies from meeting to meeting, but usually there are no more than two among the average number of fifteen participants. There is one staff nurse who has always been present. In an interview she articulated the following reasons:

"I was invited by the hospital director and chairpersons to participate in the committee and I thought [...] because that will make me think and helps keeping pace what is going to change, because otherwise, here, in this hospital you are usually the last one who knows what the people in power have decided [...]." (Ampel 2005, see Appendix 2.2.1)

The nursing director explains the absence of nurses:

"[...] we do not want to waste our time any more [...] there were so many ethical initiatives within the last years, and nothing has changed [...] we actually liked the ethics project a couple of years ago [...] but the ministers are finding nice words for unbearable situations, and we are trying to put possible solutions into actions [...] the ministers do not like to structure a real plan, they like to talk. [...] and physicians have enough stress, they go straight forward to get their work done, they are actually in a much more terrible situation than we are [...] with all these problems, most of them structural, of course [...] physicians are not used to suffering, we are, so it is harder for them [...] and I do not think that they will really participate in the committee" (Allau 2007, see Appendix 2.2.1)

In this interview, the nursing director explains how motivated the nurses had been participating in the ethics project a couple of years ago. She says that they had hopes of change with regard to a sincere and truthful communication, but as she explains, the committee work is seen as another "ethical initiative" that will not change anything. She complains that the ministers rather like to talk about problems than solving them, and that it has been the task of nurses and physicians to put things into action. In comparison to nurses, she declares physicians to be in a "much more terrible situation" due to structural problems. Although both professional groups would have to face the problems, it would be harder for physicians since they "are not used to suffering as nurses are used to" (Allau 2007). Moreover, she assumes that physicians "will not really participate in the committee" (Allau 2007, see Appendix 2.2.1).

In the *Catholic hospital* (Bach), the Ethics Committee has closed membership. Dr. Boha, the male senior physician of palliative care is the chairperson. He took the initiative to build up the committee and was supported by his superiors. Consulting the nursing director, Mrs. Beck, Dr. Boha asked Mr. Balter, the nursing leader of the elderly home as well as Ms. Bunt, the head nurse of the palliative care unit to co-chair with him. They agreed and the three people including the nursing director made a list of who to ask to join them as members (Boha 2004, see Appendix 2.2.2). The criteria for asking hospital personnel for membership were first the person's acceptance and professional respect among her or his colleagues. For Dr. Boha and Mrs. Beck it was obvious that the nursing director and the Catholic minister of the hospital (Mr. Bühler) would be committee members. While choosing persons, the aim was to get the different disciplines of the hospital as much as possible represented. Dr. Busik, the head physician as well as Mrs. Bank, the head nurse of the neurology department agreed on becoming members when they were asked. So did Mrs. Bal (head nurse of the surgical intensive care unit), Ms. Bock (staff nurse in the ambulatory care unit), Dr. Beine (surgeon), and Dr. Brecht (cardiologist of the internal intensive care unit). Moreover, Dr. Boha thought it to be a good idea to have someone as a committee member who would be in contact with a lot of people in the hospital. He could win Mr. Bier from the hospital's internal transport service (Beck 2004, Boha 2004, see Appendix 2.2.2).

The meetings of the Ethics Committee take place in a room of the palliative care academy situated closely to the palliative care unit in the modernized part of the hospital. The members meet on a regular basis every month for ninety minutes. In case of absence they inform the chairperson,

Dr. Boha in advance. The chairpersons do not take seats at the head of the table, but like all committee members they take different seats in every meeting. An interruption occurs very seldom. Members who have to react to their beepers or mobile phones always leave the room and usually come back after a short time.

During the two years of research, the membership of nurses and physicians drastically changed in the Catholic hospital. Ms. Bock left the committee after her first participation in 2005. Interviewing her to understand the reasons, she explains:

"The nursing director could convince me to become a member in the committee, but when I was sitting in the committee meeting I realized that this is not the right place for me. I cannot talk about nursing concerns with so many people. It is not that I have a hierarchy problem, but [...] I prefer smaller groups [...] about five people coming together, and at the best only nurses [...] I do not think that a Hospital Ethics Committee is a bad idea, I actually think it is a very good idea [...] but I am just not the right person there, the one who is now the member [...] I think she is much better at speaking up" (Bock 2006, see Appendix 2.2.2).

Ms. Bock explains that she did not feel to be the right type of person to participate in an ethics committee. Her colleague, Mrs. Busch, she argues, would be a nurse who would speak up. She thinks that a small group of nurses would be easier for her to talk about nursing concerns. Such nursing concerns, as she explains are "questions on the use of *living-wills* and *end-of-life* care" (Bock 2006, see Appendix 2.2.2, emphasis added).

Why did the physicians leave the committee? Dr. Beine left the hospital including the committee in summer 2006 for taking over the position of a senior physician in another hospital. This also accounts for Dr. Brecht in winter 2006. While the nurses, Mrs. Bal and Ms. Bunt, could no longer participate in the committee because of being seriously ill. Mrs. Bank made her decision to leave the committee after membership for one year and a half. She argues in the interview:

"I had to leave because the re-organization of the neurology ward took so much time that not much energy for the ethics committee was left. I hadn't expected it to be so exhausting. And [...] I am glad that I can talk about it now [...]. I thought after 20 years of nursing experience there wouldn't be anything that I couldn't cope with [...] but then the new patients of early rehabilitation taught me a lesson. The patients are very, very ill and most of them are dying, they are young [...]. I had to realize that taking care of them would be my daily job now [...] and then, in the committee we were talking about the elderly and patients' autonomy in a state of dying [...] and that there isn't anything we could do for them any more. I asked myself why do we have to give up? There is a lot you can do when you can do nursing care. You know, I was just thinking differently. At that time when the committee was talking of letting people go, I had to care for two patients who could not eat any more and there was no longer any medical intervention possible [...] but, you know, nursing care was possible, [...] good care at the end of life [...] is this nothing? To tell you the truth, the thing is, since we have this new unit of early rehabilitation and as I told you, it is difficult and time-consuming work [...] since we have this unit we are given more nursing personnel. Now I am allowed *to really care*, and this is really the best thing that could happen to me" (Bank 2007, see Appendix 2.2.2, emphasis added).

For Mrs. Bank it was important to see and experience that nursing care could still be practiced when medical intervention was no longer possible. She emphasizes that the fact of having more nursing personnel on the new rehabilitation unit allows her to "really care". When I asked her what this means in terms of practice, she explains: "Just, doing all the nursing care that needs to be done like bedding, mouth care, feeding [...]" (Bank 2007, see Appendix 2.2.2).

In sum, the physicians left to follow their career, and the nurses had different reasons: One nurse left because she did not feel that a multidisciplinary committee could be the right place (for her) to articulate nurses' concerns. Two nurses, Mrs. Bal and Ms. Bunt were no longer able to be members due to their illness, and one nurse, Mrs. Bank got into a conflict about care at the end of life that was being solved beyond the committee work: On the unit she was working, conditions changed due to more nursing personnel: She could practice "good" care for seriously ill neurology patients and the dying. Ms. Bock as well as Mrs. Bank emphasize end-of-life care as nursing concerns.

Like the hospital Bach, the Hospital Ethics Committee in the *Municipal, now privatized hospital* (Clön) has closed membership. The monthly committee meetings of this committee take place in the so called "House of the Ministers" which is the oldest building of the hospital area. The meetings usually last for two hours. The members of the committee sit around two small round tables with no assigned seats. Usually tea is served by the female minister Mrs. Carr. The male nurse, Mr. Commer and the physician, Mr. Ceisch (Commer 2005, see Appendix 2.2.3) announced themselves chairpersons of the committee. While the nurse is the first chairperson, the physician has taken the position of his deputy.

The nursing director, Mr. Cidder who is not a committee member, has supported the staff nurses to get actively involved in the ethics committee work, and bring forward "that ethical issues cannot be separated from social issues" (Cidder 2007, see Appendix 2.2.3). Three out of four staff nurses, mainly in leadership positions (head nurses on the ward) have regularly been present in their role as committee members. They are especially active with regard to participation in educational classes on "ethics" and are the ones who are engaged in taking over the role of the moderator for the retrospective and concurrent case consultations. There were two members that left the ethics committee during the time of my research: The nurse, Mrs. Calle because she was going to leave the hospital in order to finish her studies at the university and the social worker, Mrs. Clemens who left the hospital for a new job at a different one.

	Hospital Ast	Hospital Bach	Hospital Clön
Membership	Open: "Everybody working in the hospital can participate in the meetings." Usually about 12–16 people attend.	Physicians (4), Nurses (5), Ministers (2), Technical Service (1)	Physicians (2), Nurses (4), Ministers (3), Hospice Care Representative (1), Psycho-oncology (1), Retired lawyer (1), Patient Representative (1)
Leadership	Male theologian (Ethics Expert), Female lawyer	Male physician, female nurse (both Palliative Care), Clinical pastor	Male nurse (Management), Male physician (Internist)
Meeting	monthly	4–6 times a year	monthly

Table 1   Membership, Leadership and Frequency of Meetings (2005)

Looking at written papers from the outside of these committees, they did all look alike. Documents created during their design phase, like standing orders or preambles as well as the minutes of their first meetings refer mainly to membership and functions which are taken over from the US-American model. But, as the presented interviews above have shown the practices, procedures and forms of participation are strongly connected with the historical background of each Hospital Ethics Committee.

2 Analysis of the Field Data

This chapter presents my analysis of the participant observations in the practical arena. I examined the talk about selected issues of concern which were presented during the meetings (see method explained in Practical Arena Analysis, chapter one).

The dominant *issues and themes* are identified and the *way* they are discussed and dealt with is analyzed. The leading questions have been: What counts as an ethical problem? Who defines it? Which issues get attention and which ones are excluded, sidelined and dismissed? What kind of caring issues are raised by whom and what kind of responses are given? How do the different members of the committee cope with concerns of care and how much room for discussion is given to them? Do the issues which are attended to, especially issues of caring practices, change in the course of a discussion and how are they framed? What conclusions are drawn when caring issues are discussed and how are they put into action? Who feels responsible for the brought up concerns (of care) and what are the emerging conflicts revealed in the course of the discussion? More generally, the questions are not focused on how problems are properly resolved in the first place, but how problems are structured, and how the discussion on resolving the problems operate.

The chapter is subdivided into four sections which are titled according to the themes and issues that were discussed during committee meetings in all of the three hospitals. Whenever possible, in order to reveal the authentic data, I linked the identified themes and issues with the original phrases and statements given by the field actors. For example, with regard to the committees' task of policy making, it was tube-feeding that turned out to be an issue of concern for the committee members and one member called the problem "a loss of senses".

First, I will show how the committee members of the Lutheran, Catholic and privatized hospital dealt with the task of education and policy making. Then I will turn to the task of retrospective and concurrent case discussions.

Extracts of committee discussions as well the complete conversations about the cases will be presented. The subsequent excursus on a policy statement on nutritional support for the elderly can underpin the problem raised by the field actors.

Education and Policy Making:
Training, Management and Regulations

First I will give an overview of how each committee that I observed understands the task of education and policy making. Then I will contrast two different ways of how the committees practice "ethics" education. With regard to policy making, my analysis of two committee discussions will be presented. Here, tube-feeding for the elderly has emerged as an issue of concern and thus I will finish with an excursus to give information about a policy statement on nutritional support for the elderly (2003).

What are the Performances of Education and Policy Making?

How do the committee members of hospital Ast, Bach and Clön understand the task of education? Hospital Ast, Bach and Clön do not refer explicitly to education as a part of their work, but what the committee members talk about is first, a necessity to learn how to moderate "ethical cases", second, to invite "ethics experts" to give presentation on special issues like Living Wills and third, to offer and prepare "Ethics Days" (hospital Ast and Bach) or an "Ethics Evening Forum" (hospital Clön). On an "Ethics Day" usually one topic is put into focus and experts from outside are invited to present papers. The "Ethics Day" serves mainly the hospital personnel but people from outside can also be invited. While hospital Bach has an interest in reaching hospital personnel for participation in an Ethics Day or Symposium (Boha 2005, see Appendix 2.2.2), hospital Clön and especially hospital Ast want to get as much public attention as possible (Craft 2005, see Appendix 2.4.3: C 29; see also Appendix 2.4.1: A 88–91).

Although moderation of case consultations is an issue of knowledge and training in every hospital, it is approached differently. Feeling "really competent" who has undergone a training, who knows about the "experts" and who has experience is an issue of concern continuously discussed in committee meetings (see Appendix 2.4.1, committee conversation 2005: A 16–18, 2006: A 157–158, A 205; 2.4.2, committee conversation 2005: B 10–15, B 22, B 30–33, B 118).

What do the committee practices tell about policy making? Policy construction can be a very influential process as US-American literature on Hospital Ethics Committees and the expert interviews have revealed (see Historical Analysis). Especially Do Not Resuscitate (DNR) orders have mostly been a policy issue in the work of US-American Hospital Ethics Committees (Bartels 2004, see Appendix 1.2.2; Haddad 2005, see Appendix 1.2.2). Compared to Hospital Ethics Committees in the US, the members of these three committees in Germany show rather reservation and hesitation with regard to policy making. Although the head nurse of the Intensive Care Unit in hospital Bach has kept asking for regulations with regard to end-of-life questions like DNR orders since committee establishment (Buth 2004, see Appendix 2.2.2), the Ethics Committee members have continuously been postponing this issue. None of the committees in hospital Ast, Bach and Clön have started with policy making in the beginning of their work, but hospital Ast developed a draft with regard to Living Wills and in hospital Bach as well as in hospital Clön the possibility of having a policy on tube-feeding was discussed.

Education as a Training Program versus Doing one's Homework

In hospital Ast and Clön the educational program turned out to be a 'moderation training' and the question during committee meetings was: Who participates?

For three committee members (two theologians and one nurse) of the Lutheran hospital (Ast) it was possible to attend an educational program – offered by experts of ethics outside the hospital – on how to moderate case consultations. When Ms. Ampel asked the committee chairpersons for participation, she became the fourth one (Ampel 2005, see Appendix 2.2.1).

During a meeting of the ethics forum, the committee members find out that nobody from the Elderly Care department attended the moderation training. A conflict arises: The representative of the Works Council, Mr. Arloff questions whether they would have been informed. The chair, Mrs. Amt tells that everybody could show their activity to participate. Mr. Arloff gets angry and opposes: "You cannot expect any activity of them if they do not know anything about it! Was it really open to everybody? Has anyone put the concrete question: 'Do you want to take part in a moderation training?' [...]. I have my doubts" (Arloff 2005, see Appendix 2.4.1: A 24; see also for context A 22–23). The theologian, Mr. Apostel remarks that there is a need to "[...] make transparent who participates and who does not participate [...] [Since] there is always a selection beforehand" (Apostel 2005, see Appendix 2.4.1: A 92). Mr. Arloff is not convinced that the Elderly Care nurses got a chance to attend the moderation training. He mistrusts the procedure of who is informed by whom about what. Mr. Apostel even talks about a "selection beforehand".

Thinking of participation as democratization in terms of John Dryzek (see Relational Analysis, chapter three) it is unclear whether an expansion of participation with regard to the Elderly Care nurses is a collective decision. Whether their participation is "real" also arises with regard to the "Hospital Holding Conference". The director thanks the committee members for their participation in the Holding, and Mrs. Alt asks: "Are we (the elderly home) represented in the Holding?" (Alt 2005, see Appendix 2.4.1: A 155). An answer is not given, but the question rather ignored.

The privatized Municipal Hospital's Ethics Committee (Clön) is engaged in a continuous educational ethics program offered for clinicians. The chance of participation in formal educational training is a constant topic that is usually announced by the chairperson (nursing manager), Mr. Commer, in each committee meeting (Committee conversation 2005, see Appendix 2.4.3: C 9, C 32, C 49, C 133). In one meeting, when Mr. Commer is trying to motivate the committee members to attend educational classes on ethics, the committee members feel the need to give reasons why they would not be able to participate. The oncology nurse, Mr. Cüster argues that it would be impossible due to a lack of personnel at that time (Cüster 2005, see Appendix 2.4.3: C 33). The physician, Dr. Ceisch tells that it would be too much being away that week (Ceisch 2005, see Appendix 2.4.3: C 33).

Generally, in both hospitals (Ast and Clön), but most evident in hospital Clön, it is the nursing profession that mostly participates in the ethics training program. Some of the theologians and social workers have attended the training, but none of the physicians. The same acounts for the conferences on ethical issues offered by the committee. While nurses are attending conferences outside the hospital, physicians do rather hold back. In comparison to other committee members, nurse committee members in hospital Clön are the ones who have mostly participated in educational classes on ethics and moderation techniques. Therefore they voluntarily take over the role of moderating discussions during committee meetings.

According to the standing orders in the Catholic committee, the educational role of the committees consists of educating the committee itself as well as those people working in the hospital. The question who is going to participate in what kind of classes or programs has never been raised during the observed committee meetings.

Soon after the committee in the Catholic hospital had started its work, a professor of Medical Ethics and an expert on the establishment of Clinical Ethics Committees had been invited to give a talk. When Dr. Boha asks in a committee meeting, how the participants liked the talk given by the expert, they reacted as followed:

> NURSE, CO-CHAIR, MS. BUNT — To tell the truth, all what he said has already disappeared.
>
> NURSE, MS. BECK — I think as an introduction it was okay.
>
> PHYSICIAN, DR. BEINE — Was there really anything new that we did not know before?
>
> NURSE, MRS. BAL — For me it wasn't too bad to get an overall orientation
>
> PHYSICIAN, DR. BEINE —I have to say that I found it kind of strange that we had to wait for him, and when he came, then, told us that he would not have much time.
>
> CHAIR, DR. BOHA — Well, I have to agree, I really expected more [...] considering how much money he got [...].
>
> HEAD PHYSICIAN, DR. BUSIK — I think there wasn't any substance [...] I found it rather pale.

Committee conversation 2005, see Appendix 2.4.2: B 1–8

In sum, the talk given by the professor of Medical ethics was neither convincing nor worth the money and the committee members are rather disappointed by what he told them about ethics committees. This might have an influence on the discussion on how to get prepared for ethics consultation. Immediately after Dr. Busik's remark given above, the committee talk goes on as followed:

> CHAIR, DR. BOHA — *remarks* — An important question we have to clarify is whether we should already offer ethics consultations on the wards.
>
> PHYSICIAN, DR. BUSIK — *reacts* — I think yes, but we shouldn't have high expectations.

NURSING DIRECTOR, MS. BECK — *pragmatically* — What do we have to do in order to feel capable of doing it?

CO-CHAIR, NURSE, MS. BUNT — *suggests* — We could prepare ourselves by doing some studies on things that can improve our competencies, such as rules for communication skills. And I think that everybody could prepare something.

PHYSICAN, DR. BUSIK — *reacts enthusiastically* — I think that is a good idea! What I could do is prepare a paper on how to do moderations well. I could look up what kind of rules are useful.

Committee conversation 2005, see Appendix 2.4.2: B 10–14

Dr. Boha asks whether it is the right time to start ethics consultations and the first reaction is given by the physician, Dr. Busik who thinks that they should start without having "high expectations." When the nurse, Ms. Bunt suggests to prepare themselves by doing some individual studies, Dr. Busik offers to prepare a paper on moderations. Later during the meeting Dr. Boha offers to prepare another paper: A form that is helpful for requesting consultations (Boha 2005, see Appendix 2.4.2: B 22). Thus, they split up the things they think they need to know into tasks like doing one's homework.

A preference of dealing with ethics in a rather informal way is also stressed in Dr. Busik's statement: "What I would really like to see is a kind of talk about ethics in this house that is not too bureaucratic, doing it with a cup of tea [...]." (Busik 2005, see Appendix 2.4.2: B 27).

While the committees in hospital Ast and Clön show a communality by both having answered the question of education with a training program, hospital Bach is different: The members draw back on their individual (home) work and have reservations towards an expert of clinical ethics.

Policy Making as a Management of Living Wills:
"Standardization, Obligation and Cost"

The Lutheran Hospital's Ethics Committee (Ast) has now drafted a policy to provide procedures on how to handle Living Wills which were presented to the hospital's central conference to give consent for implementation (committee conversation 2006, see Appendix 2.4.1: A 138–149). When the chair, Dr. Arras hands out the draft for decision, he emphasizes that they "[...] are an obligation" and that a standardization would be of use for every hospital (Arras 2006, see Appendix 2.4.1: A 138). He is opposed by his co-chair, Mrs. Amt who remarks, that "[…] Living Wills do not always fit […]" (Amt 2006, see Appendix 2.4.1: A 139). Then, laboratory specialist, Mrs. Albor puts an obligation into questions by saying: "I have listened to a discussion on Living Wills in the church […] and there was a physician who did not uphold to a Living Will" (Albor 2006, see Appendix 2.4.1: A 140). Dr. Arras stops the arising conflict with a loud statement: "Those who offend against professional standards will have to face consequences!" (Arras 2006, see Appendix 2.4.1: A 141). Instead of having put the use of Living Wills into question, Dr. Arras continuous by talking about different forms of Living Wills and compares their length and numbers of having details (Arras 2006, see Appendix 2.4.1: A 142). The head of the hospital, Mr. All proudly remarks with regard to a comparison of Living Wills: "The Bavarian one (!) costs 3 Euro and 90 Cent whereas the Christian one (!) costs nothing! In our house it will be a donation!" (All 2006, see Appendix 2.4.1: A 143). There is nothing but astonishment to be seen in the faces of the committee participants. Nobody reacts verbally, but chair, Dr. Arras turns to the quality manager, Mrs. Aqual and asks her: "I would like to ask you, Mrs. Aqual, in what way a standardization of handling Living Wills would be possible?" (Arras 2006, see Appendix 2.4.1: A 145). The comment by the Elderly Care nurse, Mrs. Alt that "[…] standardization will certainly not do justice to the elderly home" (Alt 2006, see Appendix 2.4.1: A 146) is picked up by Mrs. Amt who remarks that this cannot be decided "now" (Amt 2006, see Appendix 2.4.1: A 147).

A managerial way of dealing with questions on Living Wills goes on when Dr. Arras points out: "It seems to be good to ask whether someone has a Living Will at the time of admission" (Arras 2006, see Appendix 2.4.1: A 148). Although "someone" are most probably patients who need to be treated in a hospital, this is not mentioned. Putting it in rather abstract terms of "someone" can help see Living Wills as a form that needs to be administered rather than being occupied with the conflicts that may evolve in patients' situations. For the nurse, Ms. Ampel it is not as clear as it is to the other committee participants that Dr. Arras "admission" only implies the administrative one. When she curiously asks whether Dr. Arras would talk about the "administrative kind of admission" (Ampel 2006, see Appendix 2.4.1: A 149) she possibly had a nursing admission in mind which is meant to ask patients for their habits and listen to his or her individual story to develop a care plan.

Policy Making as a Regulation of Tube-feeding: A "Loss of Senses" and a
"Combination of Economic and Non-Medical Aspects"

Committee member Dr. Ceisch, physician of Internal Medicine in the
privatized hospital (Clön) tried to build up a working group that would
work on policy guidelines with regard to Tube-feeding. The working group
for establishment met once and since they were not able to find consensus,
they never met again. The physician remarks: "It is a pity, I really thought
that this is important, but since we spent more time arguing with each other
than being constructive on this issue [...] we failed" (Ceisch 2005, see Appendix 2.2.3).

When the committee in hospital Bach discussed policy questions surrounding the withdrawal and withholding of treatment and nutrition, tube-
feeding became a burning issue of concern after discussing the situation of a
very thin old lady with Alzheimer's disease (Committee conversation 2005,
see Appendix 2.4.2: B 100–104). Chair, palliative care physician, Dr. Boha
points out: "A feeding-tube should make sense! When a tube is the decision, then, after three months, the team should sit together again and ask,
in which way have we been successful?" (Boha 2005, see Appendix 2.4.2:
B 105). Dr. Busik remarks: "I have heard about elderly homes who demand
that patients have enteral tubes! It has become a criteria for entrance! And
this is a scandal!" (Busik 2005, see Appendix 2.4.2: B 110). Nurse, Mrs.
Busch steps into the shared indignation by explaining: "I think there is
something going on that works like an automatism: Somebody is very thin,
maybe dehydrated and the only consequence seems to be inserting a tube!"
(Busch 2005, see Appendix 2.4.2: B 111). The increasing demand by elderly
care homes and the "automatism" of inserting tubes could be interpreted in
a way as Dr. Boha sees it in terms of "[...] the loss of senses!" (Boha 2005,
see Appendix 2.4.2: B 112) while Dr. Busik draws the conclusion: "It is a
combination of economic and non-medical aspects!" (Busik 2005, see Appendix 2.4.2: B 113).

This "loss of senses" has a double meaning: On the one hand inserting
tubes has become a senseless (without reflection) routine way of handling a
technical device when patients do not eat (enough) by mouth. On the other
hand, the senses you need to deliver nursing care in terms of giving food
by mouth to the patient (temperature, taste, amount, knowing preferences)
are no longer required and are lost as a former essential part of giving care.
Moreover, at the forefront of nursing care it needs to be considered that
eating is not to put food into somebody's body, but an act of the senses.

It is about basal and oral stimulation, manual abilities, eye sight, as well as having a comfortable and stress-free surrounding. As explained by Joan Tronto care giving means putting this actual care work into practice to meet the needs while the care-taker gets into direct contact with the care-receiver who responds to the care (see Relational Analysis, chapter two). Tube-feeding demands a technical competence of inserting first, the tube, and then continuously the fluid that is filled up in a bottle hanging at the patient's bedside. The competence and institutional conditions of using the senses to care well, including watching the patients' senses is not seen as an undelivered nursing practice and the underlying conflict between (not performed) nursing care and (substituted) technical intervention.

It can be questioned whether Health Care Insurance Companies care about the increasing number of artificial tube-feeding for old and dying people as the continuing discussion shows: The leader of the elderly care home in hospital Bach explains: "If you want to do mouth-feeding when someone has a tube, then an explanation is demanded! From a caring perspective it is, of course, better without a tube (!)[40], then you get care-level three which implies more money. Persons who are tube-fed do increasingly seldom get care-level three, usually only care-level two"[41] (Balter 2005, see Appendix 2.4.2: B 114). Thus, according to the pointed out logic in terms of money, using tubes (care-level two) is cheaper than giving care (care-level three). The attention is not given to caring for patients in the sense of assuming responsibility (see Relational Analysis, chapter two) for the caring work that needs to be done. The care for and with the individual patient who does not want or is not able to eat by himself any more, but caring for is transformed into a systematic, detached manner. The response to eating and drinking of the "cared for" as a part of the caring process is substituted by a control of the patients' weight being regulated by the amount of artificial nutrition that can be quantified.

"Sometimes I have a feeling that Fresenius[42] determines the indication for inserting tubes", Dr. Boha finishes the conversation (Boha 2005, see Appendix 2.4.2: B 115). If his feeling is taken seriously as a possible analysis for an increase of tube-feeding, then the need for food would be no more than

---

40 According to a study by G. Deitrich, J. Belle-Haueisen and G.v. Mittelstaedt (2003) *Analysis of the Actual State of Nutrition of Elderly Patients Fed via PEG Tube*, up to 13 percent of the people who are tube-fed could sufficiently be orally fed.

41 Care-level three is the highest level of care to be paid by the health care insurance company. The person has to be assessed to be very needy for twenty-four hours.

42 Fresenius is the biggest market provider of feeding-tubes.

a commodity that is kept under economic control, not as costly as direct nursing care that has been reduced to counting calories, "weight watching" and a regulation of food by tube. In addition to what Dr. Busik describes as a "combination of economic and non-medical aspects", the growing amount of people being tube-fed is also combined with non-nursing aspects and an elimination of care.

Excursus: The Policy Statement on Nutritional Support for Elderly Care

According to the Medical Service of German Health Insurance Companies, the findings of their quality assessment program in the field of community and hospital nursing showed increasing deficits. The Medical Service Community felt obliged to write a policy statement on nutritional support for the elderly (Medizinischer Dienst der Spitzenverbände der Krankenkassen 2003). All of the authors of the document belong to The Medical Service of German Health Insurance Companies. When the document was published in 2003, its content got widely accepted within the institutions of health care. The introduction states that the nursing institutions can use it as a groundwork for the set-up of "effective risk-management" with regard to nutritional support (2003: 3).

The document does not only evoke troubling questions with regard to a rather rule-learning training program, but it reveals how the perspective on elderly care is limited by medical definitions and techniques to check the elderly as if they were 'risky bodies'. The paper starts with a medical definition of malnutrition, dehydration and dysfunctional swallowing. The notion "defective" nutrition is preferred since old people would have a "disturbed" sense of being thirsty. 60 percent of the elderly living in geriatric institutions are assumed to suffer from malnutrition (2003: 12). Immobility, difficulties chewing, and loneliness are identified as *risk factors*. It is recommended that any kind of reduced weight should be assessed as a risk indicator and the regular control of weight and a detailed documentation should prevent malnutrition (2003: 48). The lack of an acknowledged standard for nutritional support as well as a lack of data which could elaborate on the problem of refusing food, is referred to, but then recommendations are only described from a limited medical perspective: Measurement techniques, laboratory tests or instruments (for example the Blandford Scale or the Eating Behaviour Scale). As an important parameter for assessing the weight of an old person, the use of the Body-Mass-Index is accentuated. And, it is emphasized that since most of the techniques proved to be too time-consuming and too expensive, the (reduced technique) Mini Nutritional Assessment (MNA) could be an alternative that would be easy to handle even by nurses.

In sum, the Policy Statement on Nutritional Support for the elderly shows how care practices are (re-) regulated and disciplined. The demanded procedures and techniques of the risk-management transform caring practices to controllable functions and can discipline the work of nursing. What is paradox about nursing here is the situation, that they directly guide and control patients by using these techniques. But then, nurses themselves are guided, and controlled by regular interventions of the Medical Service. The elderly are seen as objects of treatment procedures rather than individuals having their own habits, wishes and a will. The measurement techniques that control their bodies do not relate to them as persons, but turn them into 'risky bodies'.

Case Discussions and Nursing Issues: The Definition of an Ethical Problem and the Marginalization of Care

How do committee members understand their work in terms of "ethics"? It is not clear how an ordinary problem in clinical care becomes a bioethical problem and what the characteristics are to name a difficult situation an "ethical case" that needs to be worked on in an ethics committee. For clinicians, each day is filled with action and decision-making processes. There are practical problems of communication and organisation including value questions with ethical considerations when asking oneself whether one has exercised the activities in the right way. Yet, why are some issues and questions seen as worthy of ethical attention and others are not?

"My Understanding of Ethics"

As discussed in Historical Analysis, chapter one, according to Renee Fox, US-American bioethics had not only diverted its gaze form particular kinds of social issues and especially those that affect persons who are poor or marginalized, but it had also separated social from ethical matters (Fox 1996: 7).

When the ambulatory care nurse, Mrs. Busch first enters a committee meeting, she points out as an utmost concern, that social issues should not be cut off from ethical ones. She is shortly introduced by the chairperson, Dr. Boha by informing: "This is Mrs. Busch who will be our new participant because Ms. Bock has left." After a short break, he continues by saying: "Today we want to take time for a 45 minutes case discussion, and then we also want to go on working on the papers we introduced in February." Mrs. Busch who waits till he has finished his sentence, remarks: "Sorry for interrupting you, Dr. Boha, I would like to say something about my understanding of ethics." When Dr. Boha kindly reacts by saying: "That's fine with me", Mrs. Busch explains: "For me, ethics also includes how we interact with each other, moreover: how do we deal with *disadvantaged groups*? How do we talk with *relatives*? And [...] where do we talk with others, and who talks? Are the relatives taken seriously in their concerns?" Every committee member listened attentively, but besides Dr. Boha's rather formal comment: "Thank you very much for these impulses, Mrs. Busch." Nobody gives any kind of comments, and the meeting goes on by discussing the drafts of documentary forms with regard to case consultation (see Appendix 2.4.2: B 43–48). In an earlier meeting, Dr. Busik expressed his wish that he would like to avoid bureaucracy with regard to ethics (Busik 2005, see Appendix 2.4.2: B 27). His statement did not get any reactions by the committee members. Although there is no explicit agreement with Dr. Busik, the committee's preference of seeing and doing their work in a rather informal way is revealed with regard to educational task. Their critical attitude towards regulations is exemplified in the discussion about how to deal with tube-feeding.

Using the Warmth of a Patient's Belly: "A Petit Ethical Problem"

In the following I will present the complete conversation of the ethics committee members when they worked on a retrospective case consultation. My analysis follows afterwards.

In the beginning of a committee meeting in hospital Clön, the minister, Mrs. Carr reports, that a nurse had written down a concern in order to consult the committee. The female minister took the paper to the committee meeting and read it aloud. The nurse had experienced a situation two years ago that was still bothering her: An elderly female patient was in need of a blood bottle. When the blood bottle arrived from the lab, it was still very cold, and the physician on shift asked the nurse to put the bottle on the old lady's belly, so that the blood bottle would warm up easily for her. The nurse, who knew the patient, could not imagine doing it. The patient had been sleeping and was not in an alert condition at all. The female physician then told her to ask another nurse to do it, someone who would be more professional than her. The discussion in the ethics committee developed as follows:

MINISTER, MRS. CARR — That is really uncomfortable to get a cold something on your belly!

PHYSICIAN, DR. CRAFT — This is absurd from a medical perspective. There are, of course, other technical aids that can help to warm up blood bottles.

NURSE, MRS. CESCH — This nurse feels as an advocate for the patient, and wants to take care of her autonomy.

PHYSICIAN, DR. CRAFT — This is really a mini ethical problem!

PHYSICIAN, DR. CEISCH — I think the problem emerged from hierarchy!

MINISTER, MRS. CARR — I think they have some communication problems on the ward.

PHYSICIAN, DR. CRAFT — But this is really a petit ethical problem!

The discussion ends after some minutes, declaring that this is really a minor problem. The minister explains that she will have to talk to the nurse who has revealed her concern.

MINISTER, MRS. CARR — What should I tell her?

PHYSICIAN, DR. CRAFT — You can tell her that she did not do anything wrong within the current knowledge of practice.

PHYSICIAN, DR. CEISCH — And you can add that the problem had to do with hierarchy and failed communication. [...] Well, the more I think about it, the more I feel instrumentalized by this nurse, because this is not an ethical problem at all!

NURSE MS. CALLE — You can tell her that she did not do anything wrong, and you can tell her about the possible hierarchy and communication problem behind, but never tell her that this is no or a small ethical problem.

The meeting abruptly ends, people rise from their places and leave the room. The minister keeps sitting there and takes some notes.

Committee conversation 2005, see Appendix 2.4.3: C 17–27

The first reaction is given by the minister who states "that it is really uncomfortable to get a cold something on your belly". And this actually collides with a practice of care that does not allow putting somebody into an uncomfortable state for the use of something respectively somebody else. The lady who is ill and sleeping cannot defend herself and therefore needs protection. The physician explicitly speaks from a medical perspective that "this is absurd" and that this is not the right way to warm up blood bottles, because there are technical aids. He clarifies that this is obviously not a medical dilemma in which physicians do not know how to make an adequate decision.

The nurse, Mrs. Cesch shows empathy for the nurse who has expressed her concern. She identifies the role of the nurse who cared for the old lady as an "advocate for the patient" who wanted to take care of her autonomy. Caring for her autonomy from a nurse's understanding could mean that the patient cannot articulate herself and therefore needs protection, here given by the nurse. This is nurses' mandate. It is different from the mandate of a physician who is interested in getting a warm blood bottle for medical intervention. Nursing care for patients who are sleeping implies keeping them in a state as comfortable as possible while protecting them from disturbing noises and interventions that can be postponed like "taking the blood pressure" as well as disturbing and uncomfortable interventions like putting a cold blood bottle on their warm belly.

Although the patient is in a current state of not being able to verbally interact, the nurse sees that her autonomy still belongs to her and cannot be taken away. She uses the respect for her autonomy to justify her nursing care, namely her responsibility to take care of the patient's sleep.

When the physician defines the situation as "a mini ethical problem" without giving any reason, no questions or controversial points are raised. Why this is only a small ethical problem is left open. The physician does not feel a need for explanation, and nobody else asks for it. Then the commentaries that lack explanation go on: Physician, Dr. Ceisch declares it as a problem that has to do with hierarchy and the minister, Mrs. Carr remarks that the problem might be linked to "some communication problems on the ward". Since these are exclamations which follow after the non rejected definition of a "mini ethical problem", one could ask whether hierarchy and communication are categories that can be put under the umbrella of small ethical problems or whether they are indicators of difficult situations that cannot simply be framed as ethical. Framing them in the context of small ethical problems minimizes their potential for conflicts and understanding the situation in its complexity which, of course, can harm not only patients, but can also disrupt professional identities, here nursing care.

When physician, Dr. Ceisch repeats the remark of the physician Dr. Craft that this is a "petit ethical problem" the conversation is ended. There seems to be a hidden consensus on how much time should be spent on what kind of issues. That the discussion of the concern does not deserve much time could have been evoked by the minimization of the problem. The minister, realizing that the discussion is ending, asks the rather pragmatic question: "What should I tell her?" and the first answer is given by physician Dr. Craft, who started to comment on the concern. "You can tell her that she did not do anything wrong [...]" he authorizes the minister to tell. Does this mean that the nurse acted correctly according to a medical perspective? What are finally the criteria to distinguish between wrong and right in this situation? And, who has the power to define it?

Physician Dr. Ceisch adds that the nurse should be told that "the problem had to do with hierarchy and failed communication." What does the message signify? What can the nurse take out of this kind of analysis? This is difficult to tell because there is no explanation. With regard to interrelationships, especially in between different professions, you can narrow down and contextualize nearly everything with hierarchy and communication problems in a hospital. Physician Dr. Ceisch "feels instrumentalized" by the concern of the nurse. This is a strong reproach. "This is not an ethical problem at all!" is the explanation for his feeling. Does a talk of problems which are not defined as ethical ones instrumentalize disputants? Again, it is not clear, what counts as a "real ethical problem" in comparison to a "petit" ethical problem, or a different kind of a problem, e.g. of competence and communication? Criteria are not given. What is the legitimization to minimize the nursing concern at all?

It was the physicians who had the power to declare what counts as a "real ethical problem" and what counts as a petit ethical problem. Nobody in the group asked for an explanation why the problem is declared to be a petit ethical problem. Nobody talked about the physician who told the nurse to use the warmth of a patient's body to warm up a blood bottle. What is her part in the story? What can be said about her clinical expertise and responsibility?

The nurses' professional role is to take care of the patient's sleep. The nurse theorists Winifred Logan, Nancy Roper, Allison Tierney (2002) have developed a conceptual framework for nursing practice. One component of the model is called the "Activities of Daily Life" (ADL). Relaxing and being able to sleep is one element of these daily activities nurses have to care for. This involves having an eye on the duration of sleep, times of sleep, day-and-night rhythm, sleeping quality, rituals of falling asleep, habits, and aids to fall asleep. "Knowing the patient" means knowing his or her sleeping habits and knowing the patients' special needs to get the right kind and duration of sleep that helps them to recover and gives them comfort, especially when they are in pain and dying.

The more dependent the patient is due to the situation of illness or disease, the more comfort the patient needs. For nurses, comfort implies a moral stance, clinical knowledge, and the tangible, practical skills in which they have developed expertise.

A Problem that has no Name?: "What are we really doing here?"

The discussion presented here is a reflection on a retrospective case consultation in the Catholic hospital Bach. The Catholic hospital is associated with the elderly home, and if there is a need for an ethics consultation, it is taken over by people of the ethics committee. One past consultation is reflected during an ethics committees' meeting:

The chairpersons (palliative care physician and nurse) were asked by a nurse of the elderly care home to give consultation due to the following situation: An old lady, born in the 1920s, had not been willing either to eat or to drink. The nurses in the elderly home felt helpless and had no idea what to do about it. In accordance with the nursing personnel, the consultation team (physician, nurse and pastor) arranged a meeting with the old lady; the nurse in charge gathered.

> Dr. Boha — *recalls* — When we got to her room, in the elderly home, she was caught by surprise and asked: 'Am I ill?' 'Do I have to die now?'

> Dr. Boha — *explains* — I understand that *we*, the people coming from the hospital irritated her, because we entered her room in white clothes. We answered her question. No, we are not here because we think you are ill. We want to ask you: whether you are hungry? Then the lady explained 'It is really nice that you care about my eating, but I have never eaten much in my life!'

> Nurse, Mrs. Bunt — Then I offered different meals to the old lady, but every idea was rejected. Finally, there was one meal when she said: 'Yes'. The nurse in charge felt quite uncomfortable and said she would arrange getting the meal. Then we (consultation team) could leave.

> Nurse, Mrs. Bunt — *remarks with a smile* — I wonder what we are really doing here?

Dr. Boha — *repeats smilingly* — Yes, we should reflect this situation: what are we really doing here?

The other committee members neither asked, nor questioned anything. They were listening carefully, some of them were smiling too. Dr. Boha closes the meeting, thanks for coming and wishes everybody a Merry Christmas.

Committee conversation 2005 (see Appendix 2.4.2: B 124–127)

The nurses in the elderly home cannot cope with an old lady who is refusing to eat and drink. They are possibly afraid of letting the old lady die in case she continues rejecting food. They might also be afraid of being blamed for it, because taking care of the intake of food belongs to their professional responsibility. Since the old lady does not seem to respond to the care-givers, they probably feel unsure whether their care has been attentive enough and whether they might have overlooked something. As a way out, the nurses ask for the ethics consultation by calling the chairpersons of the ethics committee, and the head nurse agrees to a meeting with the old lady.

When the consultation team including the head nurse enters the lady's room, she is self-confident and asks her question right away. The old lady, seemingly needy for food, but without willing to eat, is the one who reveals the situation as a grotesque comedy: She is surprised that people in their professional white coats are visiting her and spontaneously asks: "Am I ill? Do I have to die now?" Since she has reached the last part of her life, dying is not that far away from her imagination. Why should she expect that hospital personnel would come over to ask her, what she would like to eat? She has never eaten much in her life, and as a matter of fact, getting older implies that the need for food and drink decreases.

The physician realizes the reason for her irritation and expresses it in the ethics committee. Both he and the nurse smile about this situation because they are irritated themselves. One question in their mind probably was, did four people really had to go to an old lady who is fully competent to articulate her needs? And, of course, the following questions are relevant to understanding the problem: What does this old lady really need? Have the nurses responded to her needs besides caring for her food? Is there not at least one nurse who knows the old lady well and knows how to respond to her? What is really known about her eating habits? How much food does she really need at that time? What is "enough" for this old lady who has not been eating much her whole life? This is not clear. Does she finally decide for a meal, because she really likes the suggested dish, or does she just want to get rid of these strange people visiting her? While reporting on this case consultation, neither the consultation team nor any other committee member including nurses raise questions of care. The only question put here is, "What are we really doing here?" This question is repeated several times, but not answered. The reaction is a smile that renders the past consulting situation into a humorous tune.

Although this behaviour, at first sight, fits the way the conflict has been dealt with, at second sight, it conceals questions of care practices and sharing responsibilities, procedures and effectiveness of ethics consultation. The ignorance of questions from a caring perspective releases the nurses of a confrontation with their professional duties and challenges the reflection on their unique conflicts of care.

Coping with the conflict of not knowing what to do because an old lady refuses eating ends up in an ethics consultation that leaves the problem a nameless one, because it turned out that at least the old lady hasn't got one. The kind of talk that is offered to the old lady by the consulting team gives insight into caring work that originally belongs to a nursing competency, namely relationship-based caring practices by knowing the patient and her eating habits. Eating as an activity of daily living is more than putting food into the body since eating and drinking imply a cultural and social meaning. Thus, not wanting to eat can have several reasons, for example, feeling isolated and lonely. I am not saying that the nurses haven't done their job well, but the context of the problem of why they finally called for an ethics consultation is not clear. Dying is something the old lady feels reminded of when the "hospital people" come in. This is obviously not something she has started deliberately. The way she reacts to people coming into her room implies also that she is prepared to listen to people telling her what to do, what she is expected to do, maybe even giving strict orders to her. During the talk with the "hospital people" she explains that she has never eaten much in her life. In fact, nevertheless she has turned quite old. From her perspective eating has never been a problem in her life. Consequently she is astonished that it should be one now.

In short, what the analysis of this part could show: Caring is marginalized, nurses are marginalized, and they further marginalize themselves as the issues of concern for them are systematically ignored: Declared to be at best, "petit" ethical problems, and not part of "what we are really doing here".

Case Discussions and Medical Issues:
Age, Isolation and Caring Responsibilities

The analysis of the data with regard to case discussions revealed a recurrence of the categories named in the headline above: Age, gender, isolation and caring responsibilities. In the following, each case discussion is presented separately in its full length and interpreted afterwards.

Old, alone and a Diagnosis of Dementia: "She wants to go home"

As announced at the beginning of the meeting, the physician of Gerontology, Dr. Ammen interrupts the meeting for a case presentation. Dr. Ammen reports:

> DR. AMMEN — A female patient born in 1928 had been treated at the Medical School, she had suffered from a de-compensated heart insufficiency, and the General Practitioner had referred her to the hospital. It turned out that she had had a heart infarct. She was referred to the hospital for rehabilitation. Her physical capacity was limited, and she did not feel safe moving. Finally, dementia understood in the widest sense was diagnosed. She was neither orientated in time nor in space. She kept talking about her wish to go home. Her brain waves showed an insufficient blood circulation. A form of vascular dementia was identified. It was realized that her home was sealed. Her neighbour had told that her flat had been absolutely run down. It had been a long time since she had allowed somebody to enter her flat.
>
> There had been the question whether she would still be contractually capable. In the hospital, she was gradually arriving at a state of being able to go home. But, she was not aware of her problems, she kept asking: When am I allowed to go home? Within the team it had been an unanswered question who would clarify things about her condition. Today, this morning, the ward informed me that she left the hospital on her own. Like every day she was going to the kiosk, but then she did not return. She disappeared! [...] Looking for her was in vain. What should I say? She is hard of hearing, suffers from diabetes, and has a walker. [...] I would like to ask the ethical question from my perspective at this point: How can patients with advanced dementia get involved in the decision-making-process? Her liability was limited, but she understood that her flat needed to be cleaned up and that otherwise she must not go home.
>
> CHAIR, MRS. AMT — Thank you for this report!
>
> *Mrs. Amt invites the committee participants to ask questions.*

Social worker, Mrs. Antenne — *asks* — What forms of incapacitation are possible?

Dr. Ammen — *reacts* — You know, the diagnosis is very complex! The medical school had treated the heart disease, but her dementia had not been diagnosed!

Ms. Antenne — *continues asking* — What about her relatives?

Dr. Ammen — *answers* — Looking for her relatives was in vain. There was no concrete address given by the patient.

Ms. Antenne — *asks* — And her General Practitioner?

Dr. Ammen — *looks astonished about this question and declares* — We did not get in contact with him.

Chair, Dr. Arras — *wants to know* — What do you think is the real problem? What do you think does it tell that she continuously articulates *I want to go home*? What is the symbolic meaning?

Minister, Mr. Apostel — *points out* — She had been probably stressed in the Medical School Hospital.

Minister, Mrs. Acker — *agrees* — Yes, I think she could not cope with her situation there.

Dr. Ammen — *explains* — We are talking about a quiet woman who only reacts if you ask something. Other patients in her condition, can turn aggressive!

Minister, Mr. Arche — *asks* — Would it not have been necessary to engage a legal guardian earlier?

Mrs. Antenne — *questions* — Is such a kind of patient not usually referred to short-term-care?

Nurse, Ms. Ampel — *asks* — What about nursing? What about nursing concepts for dementia?

Dr. Ammen — *answers* — Nurses could not do much. They (dementia patients) can be so rottenly demented that you cannot reach them any more.

Dr. Arras — *nervously states* — The question what she really wants is unclear. This is unsatisfactory.

Dr. Ammen — *explains* — The working stress has grown so much that we cannot save time for such kind of questions!

Chair, Mrs. Amt — *concludes* — I think we have to thank you for bringing in this case! Thank you very much, Dr. Ammen!

Dr. Ammen leaves the meeting and Mrs. Amt moves over to the next topic.

Committee conversation 2005, see Appendix 2.4.1: A 105–124

Dr. Ammen presents the medical history of an old lady who had a heart infarct and is diagnosed with dementia. He tells that she was neither orientated in time nor in space. With regard to social aspects, he remarks that her neighbour had mentioned her unclean flat in which she had not let anybody in for a long time. She kept talking about her wish to go home, but this remained an unanswered question for the team. Finally she left the hospital without telling anybody. When the social worker, Ms. Antenne asks about the presence of her relatives and a possible contact with her General Practitioner, the physician explains, that her relatives were not found and that nobody has yet tried to get into contact with her family doctor. This is strange since physicians usually get in touch with family doctors to get to know more about patients, especially when no relatives are present.

When the chair Dr. Arras asks what the "real problem" could be and what the symbolic meaning of her appeal "I want to go home" might be, there is no idea given. Mr. Apostel explains that she had probably been stressed in the Medical School Hospital. The question arises whether she has in any way been taken seriously in her repeated wish to go home.

The questions asked by the committee participants whether a legal guardian should have been asked for earlier as well as whether the old lady could not have been referred to short-term care are left unanswered. When the nurse, Ms. Ampel asks about the role of nursing and new ideas of how to deal with dementia patients, Dr. Ammen quite harshly answers that nurses could "not do much" because dementia patients "can be so rottenly demented" that they are unreachable. Apart from the fact that this statement implies a devaluation of people who are dement, it also shows that new ideas about how to deal with dement people are ignored. The nurse, Ms. Ampel seems to be informed about dementia care and rightly asks about the role of nurses. Since it is a professional task of nursing to take care of dementia patients according to the standards of knowledge it is astonishing that their caring responsibilities are left out in the discussion. Moreover, it could also be questioned whether the physician, Dr. Ammen comes to present the problem about a patient who ran away, and not the nurse whose responsibility it was to take care of the old lady who might run away since it is a characteristic of people who are dement. It is not the physician who takes care of a patient all day long, but the nurses. As his report shows, it is the diagnosis that is *his* competency and neither to see what kind of nursing care practices in the area of dementia might be best for this individual patient nor being responsible for its actual practice.

At the end of the conversation, the chairperson, Dr. Arras, frankly and nervously remarks that "this is unsatisfactory" since the question of what the old lady really wanted remains unclear. If you want to put it precisely, the question would rather be *why* it was not taken seriously that the old lady wanted to go home. In case it would have been impossible to let her go home, alternatives could have been considered like a nursing home for dement patients to which she could have taken her own belongings. "The working stress has grown so much that we cannot save time for such kind of questions!" is Dr. Ammen's reaction to the chairperson's remark. Although there could have been a controversial discussion now, chair Mrs. Amt closes the case consultation and expresses her thankfulness that the physician brought a case to report. Questions of conflict that are evolving here are: Can working stress release someone from asking questions that are central to seeing what the priority for the patient is? Can working stress release nurses from caring responsibilities? These questions are not given any room to be raised and conflicts of care and responsibility remain unseen.

In the next committee meeting I asked what happened to the old dementia lady and whether they would know anything about her current situation. The chair, Mrs. Amt tells with resistance: "As a surprise, she was found at home, and then she was taken back to the hospital. Soon after she died" (Amt 2006, see Appendix 2.4.1: A 204).

This astonishes the people involved since her diagnosis of dementia and her general physical status does not allow seeing her as a strong woman who has fought to get home and finally just went off. Since patients with dementia have a very strong need to move around, it is not a surprise that she walked a long distance home. There can be speculations why she was taken back to hospital afterwards. Taking the information given in the report by Dr. Ammen, she is probably declared not being able to *care for* herself. But, who really did?

A Palliative Care Patient who is Isolated and "Bleeding to Death"

A palliative care nurse requested a consultation. All facts about the situation in need for consultation were written down on a documentary form that the palliative care physician, Dr. Boha copied to bring to the committee for discussion. The documentary form (anonymous) is filled with the following questions and answers:

Who requests a consultation?
Palliative care nurse, Susan
What are the medical facts?
66 years old patient
Diagnosis: Larynx Carcinoma
Infection of tongue mouth ground in 2000, operation
Patient is bed-ridden due to weakness, tube-feeding
Main problem: Widespread throat metastasis, approx. 10x12 cm, recurrent venous bleeding from wound, with the application of haemostyptica, difficulties to reach haemostasis (2 persons are needed)
Severe pain all over cervical spine.
Patient communicates by shaking his head or nodding. There is no Living Will. During his stay here (in hospital), his wife died at home.
[...]

Table 2   Anonymous documentary form

CO-CHAIR, NURSE, Ms. BUNT — *asks* — How can you cope with the situation when he is bleeding? How much is he consciously aware about what is going on? Is he afraid?

CHAIR, PHYSICIAN, DR. BOHA — This is exactly the problem: watching how somebody is bleeding to death. Nursing cannot cope with such a situation [...] causing unnecessary pain by changing the bandage [...] And, of course, he gets an analgesia, but nurses are afraid whenever they bed him.

CO-CHAIR, NURSE, Ms. BUNT — Would it be possible *not* to change the bandage?

CHAIR, DR. BOHA — A sloughing was tried in vain, because the vessels are broken down.

PHYSICIAN, DR. BRECHT — Is he able to write? Then, one might find out what his *will* is?

CHAIR, PHYSICIAN, DR. BOHA — No, he is too weak to write. He immediately shakes his head when one enters the room. When surgeons come to change his bandage he fights as best as he can.

NURSE, MRS. BUSCH — Maybe, that is because he does not know the persons.

PHYSICIAN, DR. BEINE — I think, the nurse has a personal problem with the situation. The question is: what is unbearable for whom?

PHYSICIAN, DR. BUSIK — At home everything would be much easier [...] you can just close the door. Then, the End.

Minister, Co-chair, Mr. Balter — I think the question is: Is there any mean-
    ing in what I am doing? What is the patient's future perspective?

Chair, physician, Dr. Boha — Usually, these patients come to an arrange-
    ment for a very long time.

Co-chair, minister, Mr. Balter — Is the patient religious? What about the
    relatives?

Chair, physician, Dr. Boha — I had the impression that he is rather fatalistic
    [...] someone who is socially isolated and has neither relatives nor friends.

Committee conversation 2005, see Appendix 2.2.2: B 49–62

Immediately after the committee members have read the documentary
form, the nurse, Ms. Bunt points out the difficulty to give care to the patient while he is bleeding and possibly afraid. Physician Dr. Boha agrees
that this would exactly be the problem and that nurses cannot cope with the
"unnecessary pain" that is caused by changing the bandage. When asked
whether the bandage might not be changed, Dr. Boha tells that an alternative technique to avoid changing the bandage was unsuccessful. Physician,
Dr. Brecht has the idea that the patient might write down his will, but then
Dr. Boha explains that the patient would be too weak to write, and that
he would immediately shake his head when someone enters the room. The
nurse, Mrs. Busch remarks that this behaviour might have to do with the
fact that he does not know the person who comes in.

It seems that the committee members are looking out for good ideas
but they have difficulties finding a helpful answer to the problem. Finally,
the physician, Dr. Beine identifies the problem to be a personal one for the
nurse. For him the question is: "What is unbearable for whom?" Before
anybody of the committee participants can react to his statement, physician, Dr. Busik points out that the situation for the patient would be very
different at home: "[...] you can just close the door. Then, the End". His
thought could be that apart from institutionalized care in the hospital the
patient could take the freedom to die. After three questions and comments
expressed by nurses and six statements given by physicians, the minister Mr.
Balter interposes that the question to be raised is the one of whether there is
any meaning in what "I am doing" and what the patient's future perspective
is. He also asks whether the patient is religious and thinks of his relatives.
The physician, Dr. Boha talks about his impression that the patient was
rather fatalistic and socially isolated without relatives and friends.

Then the discussion ends and Dr. Boha who is the senior physician of the palliative care unit and therefore responsible for the patient of concern explains that the palliative care team finally decided to do only what was absolutely necessary so that the patient could feel comfortable. Since the pain had increased, the pain therapy was becoming the focus of concern. The patient did also need to be sedated, and finally calmly died (Boha 2005, see Appendix 2.2.2: B 62).

A Patient with a Head Tumour living in Isolation: "We cannot solve Society's Problems"

The head physician Dr. Anton comes after the ethics forum has already started. The meeting is interrupted so that he can report his current case of concern:

HEAD PHYSICIAN, DR. ANTON — A 45-year-old patient was at the hospital last fall. He was a strong smoker. His head tumour was not easily operated. A specimen was taken for histology examination, a moderately differentiated tumour. There had been staging, the typical laboratory examinations, sonography, and in the midst of November a combined radio-chemotherapy was ordered. The patient was discharged from the hospital at the beginning of the year. He had great difficulties swallowing and got back into the hospital. Then, a renewed staging was done. When the tube was given, it went technically well, but not for the patient: he began suffering from diarrhea and got expensive stabilizing medication. We really invested something in this young man! Then, in addition, a colon tumour was diagnosed. Surgeons estimate his chance of cure by 20 percent. What we thought about [...] is first, the question of taking him to a hospice, and second, an operation on his colon.

MINISTER, MR. APOSTEL — asks — What can you tell about the will of the patient?

SOCIAL WORKER, MRS. ANTENNE — asks — What about his social surrounding? What can be said about the involvement of his relatives?

HEAD PHYSICIAN, DR. ANTON — answers — He wants to live. There is the will to live! He lives quite isolated. Once in a while there is his [...] I think, she is his partner.

HEAD NURSE, MS. AMPEL — What about the metastasis? What can be said about his life-expectancy?

HEAD PHYSICIAN, DR. ANTON — Only a few metastases, no metastases in the bone-skeletal system. The life expectancy is about five years.

Chair, Dr. Arras informs the participants that they do want to discuss the case with the 'fish-bowl method'.

CHAIR, DR. ARRAS — *explains* — An inner circle is needed. Each of the persons who has been involved in the case, takes over his or her role. In case anybody would like to get out of his or her role, anybody else of the participants can slip into the role.

One of the participants asks for a more detailed description of the method, but no explanation is given. Then, Dr. Arras arranges the inner circle, and motivates the committee members to participate in the role play.

MINISTER, MR. ARCHE — *asks* — Where do we have to put the patient?

HEAD NURSE, MS. AMPEL — *remarks* — The position of the patient is unclear. And I think there are a lot of things unclear.

MINISTER, MR. ARCHE — Nobody really knows (!) the patient. Hospice means giving up! The patient has no hope any more.

MINISTER, MR. APOSTEL — More persons should be taken into the boat.

Silence.

Head physician, Dr. Anton asks whether he could play the role of the physician and Dr. Arras explains that he as a protagonist should not get involved in the play. Although Dr. Anton has not named any other persons while describing the case, the minister and nurse members of the committee remark that their role is possibly important.

HEAD NURSE, MS. AMPEL — I would really like to participate in the play, but what is the role of nursing here?

PHYSICIAN, DR. ANTON — The patient has been very trustful to the nurses. In comparison to the nurses, he talks very rarely to physicians. Yes, to whom he talks are the nurses.

Head nurse, Ms. Ampel takes a seat on a chair that should represent the nurses.

MINISTER, MR. ARCHE — What about a minister? What can you tell about his part?

HEAD PHYSICIAN, DR. ANTON — No, nothing. A minister has not been in yet.

Nevertheless, a minister takes a seat in the inner circle of the role play.

HEAD PHYSICIAN, MR. ANTON — *does not turn his face to the others, but looks as if he would talk to himself* — The way I (!) would handle it, is the following: if a patient has got a chance to survive, then, I will inform him, I will talk to him. If the patient does not have a chance, then, I won't talk to the patient, only, in case he asks for it. I think, you shouldn't take the hope away. Therefore, the idea of hospice, I think, is not a good one, because the patient can think you has given up on him.

I ask myself, what are we doing with the therapy. What are we actually doing? We have decided to put the missing protein into the infusion, but no other medication. He is probably going to die within the next three days. There have been discussions about a possible operation.

Chair, Dr. Arras interrupts his monologue and refers to the role play by declaring that now the participants in the role play would have the word.

HEAD PHYSICIAN, MR. ANTON — *asks* — Is this play really necessary? In reality, I am involved as a physician who treats the patient!

CHAIR, DR. ARRAS — *repeats* — This is not possible for methodological reasons!

Role-taking:

Senior physician, psychosomatic, Dr. Amso takes over the role of the head physician, Mr. Anton and takes a seat. Nurse, Ms. Ampel takes over the role of a prospective community nurse, and Social worker, Mrs. Antenne plays herself in the role of the social worker.

Role-making:

DR. AMSO — *starts* — What is the matter here is the question of dying well and having a good death.

Silence.

SOCIAL WORKER, MRS. ANTENNE — Does the patient know about this?

Nurse, Ms. Ampel — Does he know the truth?

Silence.

Dr. Arras stops the conversation by asking what the conversation team would decide on.

SENIOR PHYSICIAN, DR. AMSO — *reacts* — It is necessary to get into contact with the patient.

NURSE, MS. AMPEL — The patient needs to know his prognosis, the truth!

SOCIAL WORKER, MRS. ANTENNE — *continues the sentence* — So that the patients gets the chance to clear the things for himself that need to be dealt with.

Chair, Dr. Arras sums up the result.

MINISTER, MR. APOSTEL — *remarks* —For me this is not enough of […] attending to the patient. There is something I miss. This makes me nervous!

Meta-Discussion:

CHAIR, DR. ARRAS — *turns to Dr. Anton and asks* — Dr. Anton, what can you pick up from the conversation?

HEAD PHYSICIAN, DR. ANTON — I am astonished that the case seems not to be evident for you in the role play. What I could see is, that I might talk to the patient. *But we cannot solve society's problems!*

Minister, Mr. Apostel — *nervously* — The patient needs a roof! The central
 question is: who is the person, he trusts the most? [...] So that they would really talk for twenty minutes!

Dr. Arras stops the interruption and declares that time is running out.

Chair, Mrs. Amt — *remarks* — Thank you very much, Dr. Anton, it was very
 nice of you to present the case!

*Head physician, Dr. Anton leaves the meeting, and chair, Dr. Arras moves over to
the next topic.*

Committee conversation 2005, see Appendix 2.4.1: A 33–68

Immediately after Dr. Anton has given his medical report about the patient,
the minister, Mr. Apostel asks whether he could tell anything about the
will of the patient and the social worker, Mrs. Antenne is interested in getting to know anything about his social surroundings. Physician, Dr. Anton
answers that the patient is quite isolated and that he has the will to live. Because the nurse, Ms. Ampel asks for the patient's life-expectancy, Dr. Anton
gives the number of five years. Then the chair, Dr. Arras arranges a role play
for further discussion. The committee participants do not really understand
what they are expected to play and the nurse, Ms. Ampel frankly remarks
that not only the position of the patient is unclear, but "[...] there are a lot
of things unclear."

Although nothing is really clear about what is going on, the ministers
Mr. Arche and Mr. Apostel give comments about the situation of the patient. Mr. Arche remarks that nobody really knows the patient and sees
hospice care as giving up on the patient and a loss of hope. It is not clear
why Mr. Apostel thinks that "more persons have to be taken into the boat."
Then there is silence until the chair Dr. Arras explains that Dr. Anton as
a protagonist should not get involved in the play. Although apparently not
convinced, he puts up with this command. The nurse, Ms. Ampel explicitly
announces that she would like to participate in the play and since nurses
have not been present in the report given by Dr. Anton, she asks what the
role of nursing would be. Dr. Anton informs that the patient was very trustful to nurses and that they are ones the patient talks to. Following the rules
of the play, the nurse takes a seat.

Although Dr. Anton informs that no minister was involved in the care
for the patient, minister Arche participates in the play by taking a seat.
Then, Dr. Anton can no longer hold back what he wants to tell about his
way of informing patients about their situation: He generalizes the concrete

situation about the patient he has just talked about and explains: Patients who have a chance to survive he would talk to and patients who do not have a chance he would not talk to because then they could lose hope.

He also tells that hospice would not be a good idea since the patient could think he was given up on. While he has answered the nurse's question that the patient's life-expectancy would be five years, he is now telling them that the patient is probably dying within the next three days. It is also confusing that the medical care is reduced to putting protein into the infusion. On the one hand he thinks that transferring the patient to a hospice is not a convincing alternative, but on the other hand he acknowledges that the patient has reached the end of his life and medical intervention has become unnecessary. Hospice is first of all hospice care and does not mean to give somebody up. On the contrary, care in a hospice gives respect to the end-of-life situation and tries to go with the needs of the patient when curing is no longer possible. Thus, it could be *"curing"* that Dr. Anton has in mind when he talks about "giving up". If the patient agrees it is caring that is not stopped at the end of life. Care-giving is not only a physician's practice, but first of all a nursing practice and care for the dying has traditionally been of importance for the work of ministers.

Dr. Arras interrupts Dr. Anton's monologue and repeats that not he, Dr. Anton, but the participants in the role play would have the word. Dr. Anton puts the sense of the role play into question since it would be him who treats the patient. Thus, he underlines his authority and responsibility as a physician. Yes, with regard to medical treatment he is right in claiming his responsibility, but as revealed above, he is not the only one who is responsible for caring for the patient.

Then, the senior physician, Dr. Amso takes over the role of Dr. Anton. He remarks: "What is the matter here is the question of dying well and having a good death". He also exclaims that it would be necessary to "get into contact with the patient". Thus, he as a physician has pointed to what is missing, namely to practice care. While the social worker, Mrs. Antenne and the nurse, Ms. Ampel ask whether the patient knows the truth, the minister, Mr. Apostel thinks that there is not "enough attending to the patient". Both, the physician as well as the minister have become alert that care in the frame of contact and attending is missing.

When the chair, Dr. Arras asks Dr. Anton what he could pick up from the conversation, he tells him that he might talk to the patient. And he adds: "We cannot solve society's problems". Finally, at first sight the problem has turned out to be a communicative one for Dr. Anton. Although talking might be an important step to getting into contact with the patient, possibly telling him the truth and listening to what he wants, this is not the end, but the start of end-of-life care, provided that the vulnerable patient responds to the care given (see Tronto in Relational Analysis, chapter two). At second sight, the statement "We cannot solve society's problems" might reveal the physician's concern about the patient's isolation. He would probably like to see him dying at home and for matters of privacy and vulnerability he would rather see his relatives or friends talking and giving care to him.

Evolving Issues of Concern:
Exclusions and Questions of End-of-Life Care

As the examples have already shown with regard to the pointed out nursing and medical issues of concern, care for the dying is a central matter for committee discussions in all three hospitals Ast, Bach and Clön. The following issues of concern emerged during committee meetings and were either given room for further discussion or were excluded. In sum, the evolving issues I will present do mostly raise questions about end-of-life care, but the excluded matters of concern do also refer to more general questions of hierarchy, responsibility, institutional structure and care practices.

Excluded Issues of Concern for Committee Discussion

"To be Bound to Complicity"

A concern that is not discussed during a committee meeting in hospital Bach, but immediately afterwards while leaving the room is told by the minister, Mr. Bühler. He talks to Dr. Boha about a conflict that was reported to him: A head physician had ordered a therapy and now the senior physician and the team would be the ones to carry it out while the head physician had gone on vacation. He remarks: "From an ethical point of view the treatment is not acceptable, and the team is bound to complicity" (Bühler 2005, see Appendix 2.4.2: B 42). Then they both walk away talking to each other.

The information given here points to a conflict that has its roots in the hierarchical structure of the hospital and a division of labor: The head physician is given the authority to order a therapy that he does neither have to act out nor to take care of, but it is the senior physician and the team who were assigned to do it although they do not agree with the therapy. Whether they will accept the order is actually a different part of the process and bound to questions of comprehensibility and responsibility. The question is left open whether this issue of concern had to be talked about after the meeting and not during the meeting.

"A Patient without Perceptions"

In the committee of the Catholic hospital, the nursing director, Ms. Beck says: "There were nurses coming to me and told me about the situation that someone had declared a patient to be without perceptions, and as a consequence, the male patient was put into a room together with a female patient, and there was no partition [...]." Since there is no reaction of the chairpersons or committee members, Ms. Beck interrupts her own talk by remarking: "Altogether, these kind of cases are not that complicated I realize [...], I think I can work on them in the position as a nursing director." (Beck 2005, see Appendix 2.4.2: B 35).

Ms. Beck takes over the responsibility of dealing with the issue of securing patients' privacy due to her position as a nursing director and by declaring that the "cases are not that complicated". In her terms, complicacy defines whether an issue needs to be discussed in an ethics committee. This complicacy might surround questions of who is involved. For example, who had declared the patient for what reasons to be "without perceptions" and who reacted to this information by putting a male patient in a room with a female patient and did not take care of the patient's privacy. Even if a physician or a head nurse would have said that the patient does not perceive anything any more, the conclusions drawn are not necessarily the only ones to be done from a caring perspective. What kind of difference does the care for patients who are assumed to be without perceptions really make? Can the care about privacy be neglected for the benefit of saving room (for other patients)?

"I am a little bit Angry that our own Issues are not tackled"

That issues of concern with regard to elderly care cannot easily be brought up is specifically revealed in a dialogue during a committee meeting of the ethics forum in the Lutheran hospital (Ast). "Diaconia and Economics" is a subgroup of the ethics forum and top on the agenda. The chair, Mrs. Amt first enumerates the members of the working group and then repeats what she already explained in the meeting before (Amt 2005, see Appendix 2.4.1: A 128): "The topic is difficult to grapple. We do not really move forward. I have the idea that we can first of all profit from the research project undertaken by the University of Bayreuth" (Amt 2006, see Appendix 2.4.1: A 170). The representative of the elderly home, Mrs. Alt directly remarks: "I am a bit angry that our own issues are not tackled. We ourselves have problems to solve [...] diaconia and economy, that can have a broad understanding [...] we have to pick up something concrete!" (Alt 2006, see Appendix 2.4.1: A 171). The chair, Mrs. Amt reacts to the concern by saying: "I would like to take up that Mrs. Alt is going to make a list that tells us who has something to report" (Amt 2006, see Appendix 2.4.1: 172).

The conflict of who decides what needs to be discussed is turned into a formal secretarial solution: Making a list of persons who have "something to report". When and how by whom these textual reports of concerns will be taken as (urgent) matters to get discussed is left open. Instead, the topic of the committee conversation switches and Mrs. Alt leaves the room (Alt 2006, see Appendix 2.4.1: A 175).

"This is not an Ethical Problem"

While the topic "Diaconia and Economics" is still on the agenda in the ethics forum of hospital Ast, the following conversation develops:

Laboratory specialist, Mrs. Albor — I would like to report about the *Mafia*. It is about a discharge last week-end. The patient can no longer get his medication at the pharmacy and therefore gets it from the hospital to take home. Nurses feel being in a quandary: On the one hand it costs the house a lot of money, but on the other hand, physicians order it!

Chair, Dr. Arras — *wants to exclude this issue of concern from a discussion by remarking* — I do not want to go into this point here (in an ethics forum). The right address is the Ideas and Complaint Management Department.

Mrs. Albor — *reacts angrily* — But it has not been solved at all!

CHAIR, MRS. AMT — We will have to see how we can tackle the problem.

CHAIR, DR. ARRAS — *This is not an ethical problem!*

CHAIR, MRS. AMT — I do not agree, I think yes (it is an ethical problem).

QUALITY MANAGEMENT DEPARTMENT REPRESENTATIVE, MRS. AQUAL — *asks* — Maybe we have to take this point into the Quality Management Department? It would fit into category one: Patient Orientation.

Conversation 2006, see Appendix 2.4.1: A 174–180

While the chair Dr. Arras thinks that the "Mafia" issue[43] is not an ethical problem, the chairperson, Mrs. Amt does not agree. As Dr. Arras did before, Mrs. Aqual classifies the conflict to be an issue for the management department, but not for the Ideas and Complaint Management Department[44], but for the Quality Management Department since it would fit into the category of "Patient Orientation". She has not framed the problem as a complaint, but as an act on behalf of patients. Nobody replies to her suggestion, but then the conversation is turned back to the topic "Diaconia and Economics" by the minister, Mr. Apostel who angrily remarks that this topic has to be taken out since it would question their identity (Apostel 2006, see Appendix 2.4.1: 182).

While Mrs. Alt thought the topic "Diaconia and Economics" to be too abstract and that instead, concrete issues should be discussed, Mr. Apostel is even worried about the identity of the people working in a Lutheran hospital. Although they both put the controversial topic "Diaconia and Economics" explicitly into question, no reaction is given, but their critique is excluded.

While the issue under the headline "To be bound to Complicity" has not even been raised by Mr. Bühler (minister) during the committee meeting in hospital Bach and therefore excluded, the concern under the headline "A Patient without Perceptions" is raised and reported by Mrs. Beck (nursing director) in the meeting, but then excluded for discussion. This exclusion is actively done by herself as a reaction to the silence of the committee members after her report.

---

43 In an informant interview Mrs. Acker explains: "The term Mafia is used in this hospital to refer to all kinds of little criminal acts and in this case the nurses want to make sure that patients get the medication they really need since they wouldn't find a pharmacy that could deliver it on week-ends" (Acker 2006, see Appendix 2.2.1).

44 Ideas and Complaint Management is a separate sub-department of the Management Department that deals with complaints and ideas of how to avoid further complaints.

When in hospital Ast the participant of the ethics forum, Mrs. Alt (representative of the elderly home) announces: "I am a little bit angry that not our own issues are tackled", the kind and content of the issues referred to are unnamed and they are kept unnamed by the order of Mrs. Amt to be put on a list and hereby to get a chance to be explicated. Similarly to the concern under the headline "A Patient without Perceptions", the issue of concern "about the Mafia" is fully presented. But in comparison to Mrs. Beck, Mrs. Aqual (quality manager) does not exclude the issue for a discussion herself. The reason for the exclusion is that the chairperson Dr. Arras declares it for not being an ethical problem.

"Dying Boxes"

The following example is an issue raised in the Lutheran hospital and the repeated question is: "How do People die in our Hospital?"

Close to the end of the meeting, the chairperson of the ethics forum explains that more than three people working in the hospital had turned to him to raise the issue of care for dying people in the hospital. He explains that he does not want to ignore questions of staff members in the hospital with regard to difficulties in the care of the dying and asks the participants of the committee to name the positive as well as the negative forms of behavior towards the dying. First, the hospital director who is present at this meeting informs the committee about one observation he made.

HOSPITAL DIRECTOR, MR. ALL — A patient in bed was taken out of his room into the hall, and then a patient died in this room. Then the patient who died was taken out of the room and the one in the hall could be taken back to the room.

The director showed his surprise about this strange behaviour as he called it.

There is silence in the committee.

NURSE, MS. AMPEL — In such situations there is only one last resort, we have to put the dying patient into the bathroom. This is what we very often have to do.

NURSE, MR. ASSIS — I am glad that we do not have such kind of situations on the intensive care unit any more. When they re-constructed the unit, I had a hard time convincing the planners that we do need a separate room for people who are dying and also a room for relatives. Finally, I had to tell them that I would leave the hospital if they wouldn't do it [...] although I had just been there from Berlin [...] then they did what we as nurses wanted. We are really happy about it.

NURSE, MS. AMPEL — Yes, you can be really happy about it, but this is an exception.

MINISTER, MRS.ACKER — Since we have these room problems, we have started to attend the dying with the help of *Dying Boxes*!

The committee members (including me) look astonished when the name 'Dying Box' was dropped in. The female minister realizes the astonishment.

MINISTER, MRS. ACKER — A *Dying Box* is a box with a candle, a tablecloth and a prayer written on a piece of paper. This is what we can simply grab when somebody is dying, and this is what we can do [...] at the least.

NURSE, MRS. AMPEL — We have the problem on our ward that we usually do not know who is the responsible physician for a patient who is dying in pain. Sometimes it takes me many hours to find him!

MINISTER, MR. APOSTEL — We have a chapel and we could put the people there when they have died. Then there is room where the relatives can say goodbye.

MINISTER, MR. ARCHE — But this counts only for the ones who have already died, we are talking here about the ones who are not dead yet, they are dying!

MINISTER, MRS. ACKER — I think this is really a bizarre situation when dying people are pushed into the bathroom. Imagine you are a relative and then you are sitting in a bathroom when your loved one is dying.

The male chairperson is watching the time.

CHAIRPERSON, MR. ARRAS — I think it is best to establish a working group that will tackle this issue further.

NURSE, MRS AMPEL — This has something to do with administration! And this has something to do with physician practitioners with hospital-cottage affiliation.

The female nursing director has not participated up to this point. She looks nervous and furious.

NURSE DIRECTOR; MRS. ALLAU — What can we do and actually change in a working group when there are only nurses and ministers? Nurses cannot solve the problem!

HOSPITAL DIRECTOR, MRS ALL — This is a matter of diaconia!

There is a short silence.

CHAIRPERSON, MR ARRAS — Time is running out, we have to postpone the issue to the next meeting!

Committee conversation 2005, see Appendix 2.4.1: A 69–85

The discussion reveals the phenomena of invisibility and the unsaid. The issue of care for the dying is not on the agenda. The issue of concern has been approached by hospital staff who are not present at the committee meeting. Since this committee has an open forum they could have raised the issue themselves. Why they chose this indirect way of getting the caring issue discussed can only be answered by speculation: They feel that the chairperson is in a more powerful position. He is in a leadership role and he is also a highly respected theologian in the field of bioethics. Due to this authority the issue of care for the dying might get attention and be taken seriously. Another structural reason might be found in a simple lack of time.

The issue is not put on the agenda, but the chairperson raises it at the end of the meeting. This handling gives the impression that he feels a duty to tackle the issue somehow and at some place, but not as an official point of discussion. Since the agenda is sent out via intra-net in the hospital, this issue as an official matter of discussion could have had the following consequences: (1) People who are involved in the care of the dying could have felt motivated to participate in the meeting; (2) it could have given rise to the possibility to prepare oneself on this issue for the meeting; (3) staff who had originally raised the issue could have been informed that their concern was actually given attention to. Care for the dying then would have been a visible concern with a readable line on a piece of paper that would have taken official space and time. But instead, there is silence.

When the chairperson starts the discussion, he asks the committee participants to distinguish between the positive and the negative forms of behavior towards the dying, but as the course of the discussion reveals, except one remark by the intensive care nurse, nobody can talk about the "positive behavior".

The hospital director starts giving an example of "strange behavior" he has observed. He does not say who took the patients back and forth to the room. Usually this is work done by nurses, but he does not say it. Maybe he wants to make the situation as neutral as possible so that nobody should feel directly addressed. The question is, what could have been the kind of alternative to the described "strange behavior"? This is answered by a nurse who possibly felt she was addressed. She talks about "the last resort" for the dying: The bathroom. Hereby, she has explained the mode of behavior with a problem of space: Is there room for the dying? If not, either they have to take the dying to a place of somebody else or they have to put the dying into the bathroom.

The intensive care nurse, Mr. Assis remarks how glad he is about having the necessary space for dying patients as well as for their relatives. He had to fight for these rooms and finally was successful after he threatened to leave the job he had just got. Of course, this is not a convincing argument based on professional nursing care competence and responsibilities, but rather a strategic threat. What are the (nursing) standards in the care for the dying? Are they disregarded or have they not been established in the hospital yet? Is dying in dignity an issue that goes without saying? These questions are not a matter of the discussion.

When the female nurse, Mrs. Ampel declares the situation on the intensive care unit as an exception, the female minister reveals how the hospital ministers solved the problem: They invented a *Dying Box*.[45]

When the box is mentioned, the committee participants are astonished. Most of the people seem to have never heard about it before.[46] Nobody seems to know what the meaning is and what is inside the box. Although this name could make you think of somebody who is dying in a "box", nobody reacted on its possible connotations. Not only the talk about the "box", but also the name itself has a symbolic meaning: The *Dying Box* is a black box since nobody knows what is inside. Moreover, there is no visible shared understanding about the practice of care for the dying.

The nurse, Mrs. Ampel continues to complain about unclear responsibilities. She remarks that it takes nurses' time to find the responsible physician for a dying patient in pain. Besides the question of responsibilities, the care for people in pain is another issue raised, but not discussed further. Mr. Apostel, who seemed not to have listened to the problems just raised, talks about the chapel that could offer a place for the people who have died. His colleague tells him that this is not an answer to the problem they are facing.

The female minister, Mrs. Acker takes up the fact anew that people are dying in the bathroom. She challenges the committee members by putting them into the role of relatives who might sit in a bathroom when their "loved one is dying." Hereby, she is trying to show the impossibility of the

---

45 A week later I got to see this "dying box" in the hospital. I met a minister in the Lutheran hospital and she took a little Bible-sized wooden box out of the cupboard. She opened it and took out a dark-white candle as well as a dark-white tablecloth, and a little piece of paper with a prayer written on it. She told me that the ministers of the hospital had decided to have such boxes for the hospital on each unit in order to be able to attend to the Dying.

46 Some people seem to know something, but they do not talk about it.

situation, mainly from the emotional perspective of a relative. Putting one-self into the perspective of the patient, one would have to imagine oneself dying in a bathroom. Here, the impossibility has reached such a dimension by violating a person's dignity that the question is probably beyond the powers of imagination and therefore not asked despite its reality.

The male chairperson, Dr. Arras who is watching the time does not leave the female minister's remark to any reactions by the participants, but thinks it is best to tackle the issue by the establishment of a working group. There is a German saying: If you do not know how to go on, then establish a group who will work on it. This solution is in fact, not taken seriously, at least not from a nursing perspective. The nurse, Mrs. Ampel reacts first to this suggestion. Instead of picking up the idea, she wants to put the attention back to reasons of the problem she had referred to earlier in the discussion. Repeatedly, as it happened before, her concern is not picked up. However, the nursing director raises her voice for the first time during the meeting and takes up a position on the question of what could actually be changed in a working group consisting of nurses and ministers. Hence, she questions the power of nurses and ministers in resolving the problem. Her reaction can be explained on the following background revealed in an interview:

There had been more than one working group established to cope with the deficits of care for dying people in the hospital. Those groups were most-ly attended by nurses and ministers. And:

"There had also been a separate nursing group activity who developed a standard for the care of the dying. But, nothing got implemented [...] we are giving up" (Al-lau 2005, see Appendix 2.2.1)

When the nursing director finishes her stance (in the committee discussion) with the exclamation "Nurses cannot solve the problem!" the hospital director reacts determinedly by claiming, "This is a matter of diaconia!" By making it matter of diaconia at this point of the discussion, caring as a professional practice is reduced to a religious service. It appeals to the nurses' conscience and is morally laden. Thereby, he excludes the explanation that nurses are being impeded in their care for the dying. The male chairperson, a theologian, reacts as if this is asking too much of him, and closes the meeting without any substantial comment or outlook on the controversy.

Conflicts over care for the dying are related to spatial problems. Responsibilities are moved away from professional groups and individual persons because they have been feeling powerless to solve it. Their suggestions for solving the problem have not been put into action, but instead, have been answered by starting a second or third working group that should face the problem anew. Solving problems by ethical discussions and not by deeds has been frustrating for the nurses and ministers in hospital Ast. Therefore, the nurses do not see any sense in participation in the committee work.

Pain, Space, Nursing Shortage and Dying in the Shadow of the Palliative Care Unit

A lack of room for dying people is a problem articulated in all three hospitals ethics forums. I will first present a discussion of hospital Clön that also shows a circle of issues of concern around the care for patients in pain, nursing shortage and the question whether a palliative care unit could solve the problems. Here, I will pick up the inherent critique about palliative care as an answer to the pointed out problems about end-of-life care by presenting a short dialogue on palliative care that is taken from a committee conversation in hospital Bach.

In the beginning of the committee meeting in hospital Clön, the minister, Mrs. Carr is upset.

MRS. CARR — *recounts* — Last week I was on a ward and observed a patient who was very much in *pain*. She was in a state of dying. She was comforted. She had monstrous pain. The relatives were hanging in the chairs. You know, nowadays you can go to the railway-station and you will find somebody to get dope, but in the hospital you have to suffer from severe *pain* [...] I am still furious.

NURSE, MR. CÜSTER — We have increasing problems of getting patients in. Recently a patient was dying in a three-patient-room. We had to care for the dead body in the bathroom.

NURSE, MRS. CESCH — What do you need?

NURSE, MR. CÜSTER — *Rooms!*

NURSE, MRS. CESCH — We should get people from outside who can sit with the patient when he or she is dying.

PHYSICIAN, DR. CRAFT — We have money in the circle-of-friends cash-desk!

NURSE, MR. CÜSTER — We simply do not have enough staff, but it meets the planned number given by management.

PHYSICIAN, DR. CRAFT — The circle-of-friends does not want to sponsor what originally is the task of the hospital.

PHYSICIAN, DR. CEISCH — On the week-end I experienced that on a ward with thirty-four up to forty beds there was one registered nurse and two student nurses. Nobody can handle such a situation. How can you go home and think your work is done?

Mrs. Carr takes out a poster that she has brought over from another hospital. She opens the poster to the committee participants. It visualizes how a palliative care unit works and can be integrated into a regular hospital.

MINISTER, MRS. CARR — That is the way how it could work!

PHYSICIAN, MR. CEISCH — You cannot finance it with the money from the circle-of-friends. That wouldn't be enough.

MINISTER, MRS. CURZ — The nurses are told that they should not put forward too much *social romanticism*, then everything works out! I think it is really necessary that we tell the employer what is really impossible to handle!

Committee conversation 2005, see Appendix 2.4.3: C 134–145

The meeting starts with the female minister's, (Mrs. Carr) report about a patient who was suffering from "monstrous" pain while her relatives gave her comfort. Mrs. Carr tells how angry she is and remarks with cynicism that it would be easier to get a pain-killer ("dope") at the railway station than getting it in a hospital (C 134). The nurse, Mr. Cüster does not pick up the problem of patients in pain, but tells about the patients who are dying in the bathroom since there weren't enough room (C 135). Although Mr. Cüster tells the committee that he would need "rooms" (C 137), the nurse, Mrs. Cesch suggests having "people from the outside who can sit with the patient when he or she is dying".

The problems have shifted from pain to rooms, and then over to a recruitment of people from *outside* the hospital who should take care of the dying *inside* the hospital. It is not clear *why* nobody – besides the relatives – takes care of the people who are in pain and the obvious structural problem of a lack of rooms for the dying develops to the discussion of persons who should sit with the patient. That there are neither rooms nor people to care for patients at the end of life gets clear when Mr. Cüster remarks: "We simply do not have enough staff". And he adds "but it meets the planned number given by management" (C 140). Thus, a different type of problem is evolving: According to the logic and rationalities of personnel management the number of staff taking care of patients is sufficient but within the logic of practice, the "planned number" of staff neither meets the needs of the dying nor the demands of professional care.

The physician Dr. Craft suggested that the circle-of-friends might give money so that people from outside of the hospital could sit at the bedside of the dying patient, but after Mr. Cüster's statement, he explains that the circle-of-friend does not want to sponsor what originally is "the task of the hospital" (C 141), that is, to secure enough staff.

Physician Dr. Ceisch exemplifies the nursing shortage by telling the committee that only one registered nurse and two student nurses were on shift on the ward with more than thirty beds. Then Mrs. Carr takes out a poster that shows how a palliative care unit can be integrated into the hospital. She remarks: "This is how it could work" (C 143). Mrs. Carr obviously understands the model of a palliative care unit as a solution to the problem. She is right in probably thinking that a palliative care unit would mean first, to have more room for the dying, and second, more personnel to take care of each patient's individual needs, especially with regard to professional pain alleviation. But, beyond the question of financing that Dr. Ceisch points out, I question: Does palliative care really solve the problems of nursing shortage? And, should all patients who are suffering from pain and patients who are dying be put on the palliative care unit? Then, the spatial and staffing problems would be reproduced.

While talking about the possibility of a palliative care unit, the minister, Mrs. Curz furiously remarks that the nurses are told not to put forward too much "social romanticism" and then things would work (C 145). What could be the meaning of this statement in the context of talking about palliative care? Both, palliative care and nursing care favor a holistic approach to patient care, both emphasize the relevance of being in contact with the patient, considering his or her biography in making decisions and pay special attention to the surrounding when giving care. But, when the idea of palliative care is discussed the reproach of "social romanticism" does not come as easy as it comes when nursing ideas are discussed.

In the Catholic hospital the palliative care unit is a special place that meets all kinds of quality criteria for a human way of dying: friendly, well equipped rooms, physicians who know about pain relief, and enough nurses who have time to care. Therefore it has been a repeated matter of concern that is put into the following question: "How do people die on *normal* wards?"

At the beginning of the committee meetings everybody is invited to talk about cases or concerns he or she has been involved in or came to know by somebody else. The physician Dr. Busik starts the committee meeting with the following concern:

DR. BUSIK — We cannot assume here that everybody has the luxury the palliative care unit has. If we want to be fair, we have to see it as a problem that there are more or less ugly rooms where patients are dying in, and sometimes they do not even have a washbasin!

DR. BOHA — I think this will certainly change when renovations are done.

Ms. BUNT — I know that there are more problems around the care for the dying, nurses have told me several times [...]. Sooner or later we have to work on these questions here!

Dr. Boha heads to the next topic on the agenda.

Committee Conversation 2005, see Appendix 2.4.2: B 117–119

The idea that palliative care cannot be the answer to the problem of end-of life care is shown in the critique by Dr. Busik who declares the palliative care unit to be "luxury" for some people in the hospital while other patients are dying in very uncomfortable rooms. When Dr. Boha reacts to the statement by referring to renovations that "will certainly change" the situation, the problem of care for the dying remains being framed in a spatial and aesthetic dimension (to change from "ugly" rooms to 'nice' rooms). That is not all to say about the problem is pointed out by the nurse, Ms. Bunt. She reacts to the points of spatial and hygiene deficiencies by declaring that nurses had told her "there are more problems around the care of the dying". Nevertheless, she does not talk about these problems but says that they need to be discussed at a different time.

3 Summary

The aim of the finishing part of the practical arena analysis is to resume the findings by a summary that does not only capture the results of the data analysis, but tries to draw a cross-section by focusing on the commonalities and differences of the three hospitals. To complete the picture, some findings beyond the analysis in chapter one and chapter two are added.

The practical arena analysis in Germany shows that Hospital Ethics Committees are both embedded within the institutional structure of a hospital, its individual culture and historical background. In hospital Ast the committee was initiated as an answer to solve problems of communication being identified in a forerunning "ethics projects". Hospital Bach felt motivated to have an ethics committee due to conflicts about end-of-life care and along the establishment of the "new" palliative care unit, the idea was growing. In hospital Clön the committee was built up on the basis of an interdisciplinary working group, called "quality management and pastoral care", and this along the process of privatization of the hospital.

The name "Open-forum Model, Round Table – Dialogue Ethics" in hospital Ast that should officially allow everybody to participate and open for talks, turned out to be a misnomer since the arrangements were rather the opposite. The number of people capable of participating was expanded for collective tasks of the ethics forum and the scope of bringing more issues and areas under democratic control (see Relational Analysis, chapter three) was marked out by five subgroups that were working on selected issues. When concerns beyond the subjects of the working groups were going to be brought up, they were either referred to management, to an expert for communication problems, or set on a list (see Practical Arena Analysis, chapter two and Appendix 2.4.1: A: 25–27). The focus on nurses' participation revealed that their experiences of dealing with an "ethics projects" in the past of hospital Ast had decisively influenced their interest in attending the ethics forum. Since this project did not help to face the problems they were coping with, they were becoming quite hopeless that the work in an ethics committee would be worth it. Nevertheless, one female staff nurse and one male staff nurse were nearly always present at the meetings of the ethics forum. They were actively involved in committee discussions (see Appendix 2.4.1; Practical Arena Analysis, chapter one and two) and before the female nurse left the hospital to work in a hospice; she became one out of four chairpersons (see Appendix 2.4.1: A 209).

The committee members in hospital Clön were actually sitting around "round" tables and the starts of the meetings were generally characterized by bringing in whatever the participants were concerned about. The chairperson did not necessarily open the discussion. The ministers, physicians, nurses, hospice care representative, social worker, psycho-oncologist and a retired lawyer as well as a patient's representative discussed "cases" and evolving conflicts during meetings and had no working groups. Hospital staff brought in their issues of concern either by informing one of the committee members or by attending a meeting. In some meetings that I observed, the discussion about conflicts developed to 'circles of concern' and the decision-making was postponed to the next meeting (see Appendix 2.4.3: C 121, C 192). Nurses did not only participate in number, but with activity. Most of the committee members that attended educational 'training' programs were nurses and most of the time they were moderators of committee case consultations. Only one nurse left the hospital and the committee to finish her university studies.

While hospital Clön performed a rather informal style of committee work compared to hospital Asts' rather formalised working arrangements, hospital Bach cultivated an informal way of dealing with committee functions (see Practical Arena Analysis, chapter two; Appendix 2.4.2: B 27) as well as leadership acting. The committee members gave room to discuss shared issues of concerns and in the beginning of each meeting, the chairperson asked for "the news" to share and discuss in the meeting. The nurses I observed in hospital Bach, were active participants and one member became co-chair. A remarkable number of the nurses left the committee in hospital Bach during the time of my research. While most of the nurses left for reasons of illness, one nurse could not identify with the committee work, and another one left due to reasons of overload combined with a conflict she had during a committee discussion.

On the whole, the atmosphere and style of communication among committee members that I observed differed from a rather restricted, closed and controlled one, to a rather relaxed, open, and contentious one. The more restricted discussions were, the more the talks turned out to be difficult and broken. The more open the conversation developed, the more concerns were picked up and less questions were cut off. While in the ethics committee of hospital Bach and Clön, interruptions occurred very seldom, in the ethics forum of hospital Ast it happened that there were constant disturbances by answering cell phone calls (Committee conversation 2006, see Appendix 2.4.1: A 131 – A 204). The speed and volume of talk and in general, the committee work, in these three hospitals differed highly: In hospital Clön, the volume as well as the speed of talking to each other moved up the more issues evolved apart from the agenda; in hospital Ast, the participants of the ethics forum worked very busily on the topics of the agenda and the speed of talking was comparatively high to the committee of hospital Clön and differed extremely to hospital Bach. In hospital Bach the work and talks went rather slow and smoothly.

Using John Dryzeks' terms (see Relational Analysis, chapter three), nurses' participation appeared to be "real rather than symbolic" in the committees I observed. Compared to the US-American studies on nurses' participation, which show that nurses participate most in discussions that pertain to retrospective case consultations, the nurses of this field study in Germany were interested in education. Nevertheless, one of two actively participating nurses in hospital Ast, and more than half of the committee members in hospital Bach resigned from participation during the time of this field research.

In two of the committees that I observed, (hospital Ast and Clön) the function of education was performed as a training program, mainly to learn how to moderate case discussions and how to approach an ethical conflict by a principle-based approach. In hospital Bach education was performed in an informal style by drawing back on competencies of the members who would prepare papers on what the committee needed to know.

Policy making was generally seen as something tedious and difficult to put into action. In hospital Clön, the initiative of the senior physician who wanted to establish a working group that should work on policies with regard to tube-feeding, came to nothing and since then, further activities stopped. In hospital Ast and Bach, policy questions emerged around the issues of Living Wills and tube-feeding. When the discussions developed, Living Wills and tub-feeding were discussed in terms of management and regulation. While the chairperson of the ethics forum in hospital Ast was ambitious in bringing forward Livings Wills in the form of a standard and in terms of a professional obligation, the participants were not convinced about standardization and raised questions with regard to physician's responsibility and practical implications. Like Living Wills, tube-feeding was an issue of concern in every hospital. In comparison to hospital Ast and Clön, the actors of the field research in hospital Bach discussed their concerns about tube-feeding in depth. They were enraged by Health Care Insurance Companies that would not act on behalf of patient care but rather on behalf of market-driven principles.

The ambition of each committee was to advise on cases. All the issues of concern brought in by physicians were reported in a medical language that is characterized by a specific terminology that can do without complete sentences (see for example Appendix 2.4.2: B 49) but, when the committee discussion on the case reports developed, not the medical facts were of interest and decisive, but social questions and conflicts of care and responsibilities. Taking care of patients and giving care to patients with regard to their sleep, eating habits, alleviation of pain and questions of end of life were nursing issues of concern. The cases presented showed that the delivery of care was impeded by structural conditions and physicians' orders that would not meet nursing standards of expertise and their moral understandings of care. Moreover, due to the data, questions could be raised whether limits or even a lack of practicing care resulted from a lack of nursing competencies and responsibilities.

As the case discussions revealed, care for people who are dying in the hospital is a central matter for committee participants in all three hospitals. While concerns about dying were implicitly brought up during case discussions, the struggling questions about end-of-life care emerged beyond the agenda of the committee meetings.[47] In hospital Ast, responsibilities *who* would care for the dying *when* and *where* were unclear between physicians and nurses while the ministers found a pragmatic solution by having ('tool') boxes in stock that contain (last) aid to meet spiritual needs at the end of life. The spatial problem to care for the dying is also a matter of concern in hospital Bach and Clön. Although hospital Bach has a palliative care unit it becomes clear that not "… everybody has the luxury" to die comfortably. In hospital Clön, not only the spatial problem, but also thoughts about *who* cares for the patients in pain are aroused. Moreover, nursing shortage comes up as a burning issue for all committee members. While the chairperson in hospital Ast suggests to establish a working group that should think about

---

47 See Appendix 2.4.1: Amso 2005: A 56, Arras 2005: A 69 and 129, Ampel 2005: A 71, Arik 2006: A 236; 4.2: Busik 2005: 117, Bunt 2005: B 119; 4.3: Ceisch 2005: C 85, Cesch 2005: C 92, Carr 2005: C 135.

standards with regard to care of the dying, the chairperson in hospital Bach refers to the renovations of the rooms that would change the situation. The committee members in hospital Clön suggested inviting a person of hospital leadership since this would be the only way to begin solving the problem of a lack of nurses and palliative care. In general, when it comes to the questions about end-of-life care, all committee members in all three hospitals share their concerns. The discussion turns into a debate that provokes questions and statements for all professions.

Not in hospital Clön, but in hospital Ast as well as in hospital Bach, some issues that are raised during the meetings were excluded, either by not framing them as an "ethical problem", putting it on a list for eventual further discussions, being just silent when an issue is raised, or, by bringing it just not into the committee, but give preference to raising a concern after the meeting. These excluded matters of concern refer to questions of hierarchy, responsibility, and institutional structure as well as care practices in general.

In terms of money, for example, with regard to financing the communication training or an educational training on moderation, the ethics forum in hospital Ast is silent. Sometimes "costs" are mentioned, for example with reference to the use of Living Wills. In the ethics committee of hospital Bach, questions of money are discussed as soon as they arise, but amounts are only hesitantly given. In hospital Clön, matters of money are regularly involved in committee discussion, especially with reference to the financing of an educational class on ethics, but also in the context of the idea whether to establish a palliative care unit or not.

Résumé

In the Historical Analysis I analysed the *historical shape* of Hospital Ethics Committees. They are both embedded within and take their intellectual and moral direction from the emergent discipline of bioethics. Moreover, ethical decision-making processes by committees can even be traced back to the 1920s in several countries as well as to the invention of Institutional Review Boards. As US-American social scientists have shown bioethics was and still is developing as a theoretical as well as a clinical discipline constructed in the 1960s by professionals from various fields who have combined analytical philosophical ethics with law. I could identify the development of Hospital Ethics Committees as a *conglomeration of driving forces* and not as a response to technological progress. On the one hand, the growth of these local committees resulted from individual fates that got public attention by the work of media, turning them into eventful dramas like the Karen Quinlan story and the "Baby Does' Cases". On the other hand, their acceptance was supported by government to prevent that decision-making about living or dying at the bedside would turn into a regulation by law. Consequently, the committees served the institution of the hospital and could protect the authority of physicians. Finally, the establishment of Hospital Ethics Committees was pushed by the Joint Commission on the Accreditation of Health Care Organizations that demanded hospitals to have some structure available to deal with ethical problems arising in clinical work.

US-American nursing academics have been discussing and studied the *participation of nurses* in Hospital Ethics Committees since the 1980s. They found that nurses are members of these multidisciplinary Committees, but that their unique issues of concern find a better place in Nursing Ethics Committees. Such committees that focused exclusively on nursing issues, were first established in the form of informal working groups and developed as a parallel rather invisible movement to Hospital Ethics Committees. At that time, discussions in US-American Hospital Ethics Committees were mainly moderated by ethics experts and framed by an analytic model of a principle-based ethics which was especially criticized for its lack of narrative. Feminists with an academic background in education, philosophy and nursing have criticized that focusing on justice and autonomy can divert the attention from the patients' needs and vulnerability. An ill and dying patient is after all in a situation of being dependent on somebody else.

In the 1990s, feminists, especially those with a background in political science have worked on ideas to understand care as a social practice and the question is raised, whether anybody can be excused from being irresponsible, including politics. I have tried to develop their ideas for this research. Their refined understanding of care helped to find a language for the analysis of the field data, that is to say, what clinical caring practices are about and what the conflicts are. In the specific field of clinical care work of nurses and physicians, but also in a broader sense, care can be defined as *practices of responsibilities* that demand competencies in clinical medicine and nursing, and responsibilities that move beyond the professional (institutional) level.

The start of establishing Hospitals Ethics Committees in *Germany* goes back to an initiative by the German Lutheran and Catholic Church Association in 1997. A brochure was published that encouraged building up these local committees according to the US-American model. In German publications, the individual fate of Karen Quinlan is what is taken as their historical starting point. Technological progress is seen as a reason for the need of clinical ethics. German hospital committees have continued to develop as *a re-make of the US-American model*. At the time of my writing, as once in the USA, accreditation processes are speeding up the number of Hospital Ethics Committees. There has not been any governmental intervention yet, but last year (2006) the German Physician's Association published a call to establish Hospital Ethics Committees and strongly recommends the formulation of standards. Who is going to be in charge of and involved in this process has not been pointed out and questioned yet.

The field study in three German hospitals has revealed three different case stories about the establishment of an ethics forum and how they developed within the next two years. In terms of participation, nurses proved to be active committee members that represented various nursing expertises of the hospital, had leadership roles and developed to chairs or co-chairs of the committees. Nevertheless, they rather held back in bringing forward *conflicts of nursing*, or evolving issues of concern were *marginalized* as well as ways of exclusions took place. The nursing issues of concern that were brought in for committee case discussions revealed conflicts in delivering caring practices, such as watching patients' sleep in quantity and quality, protecting the dying from uncomfortable actions, and finding out the patients' eating habits, but were not seen as such. Instead, the committee discussion within the framework of ethics brought it up as a "petit ethical problem", thus minimizing its importance for attention and consideration. What counts as an ethical problem is part of committee discussions and belittlements as well as exclusions are made. For nurses as participants in the committees, social issues are included in the definition of an ethical problem.

The committee talks varied their affinity to (ethical) principles, medical facts, and matters of management, legal authority, and personal experiences. However, in the process of nursing and medical case discussions as well as during debates with regard to policy making, concerns about caring practices and (social) responsibilities emerged. The conflicts referred to spatial, personnel, social and caring issues. In general, the committees preferred finding new rules and standards as a response to the pointed out conflicts. But, this answer was driven either by the chairpersons or the ones being trained in "ethics" moderation (as ethics experts), and not by committee participants, that is to say, not by the ones who are acting at the bedside of the patient.

Patient care reviews that were set on the agenda and then brought in, or left out and the evolving issues of concern that were excluded, postponed, or finally successfully raised for a debate, as well as the debates on policy issues, on the whole, all of them refer to questions of care. There were physicians in the committees who would follow questions in the format: "What were the reasons for or against stopping treatment?" Notwithstanding, the underlying questions referred to end-of-life care, palliative care, elderly care, long-term care or chronic care (dementia). These 'troubled and silent voices of care' as I have tried to describe them (2006), mostly surrounded end-of-life care. The problems of having neither rooms, nor nursing personnel to care for the dying, was mostly brought up. It unfolded to be unclear who is responsible for delivering end-of-life care and how the conditions should be changed by whom. Hereby, palliative care was discussed as an answer to the problem, but was not only understood being "impossible" due to financial reasons, but proved to be part of the problem, since the "nice rooms" and being cared for well on a palliative care unit would divert the attention from "ugly rooms" and nursing care problems on other units of the hospital. It was seen critically since it would only serve some of the dying patients in a hospital.

What is the trouble with the silent voices of nursing care? What I can see in my field data is, that *not* telling the nursing problems of care means that they remain unknown for the other committee participants. But, of course, it does not mean that there are no nursing conflicts of care beyond the scope of the discussion. On the contrary, there might be nursing conflicts of care that are rather difficult to talk about, or it might be even impossible to put these kinds of problems into a language of speech. From a nursing perspective, especially care for the dying is after all care giving to meet bodily needs, and, talking about this activity exposes not only the dying patient in a state of utmost vulnerability, but also the work of nursing including its messy necessities.

Re- visiting the findings of Patricia Flynn's field study of Hospital Ethics Committees in the United States (see State of the Art, chapter one), in comparison to my findings of German hospital committees, the following can be shared: "Having a committee to discuss bioethical issues implies that ethical issues will be discussed. [...] In fact, this is not true" (Flynn 1991a: 182). Moreover, the observation can be shared, that in committee discussions there is much that is simply not picked up, but rather cut off, and there are more questions than responses and a variety of interruptions. But, what cannot be agreed on, is: "The advice requested, and decisions made, are framed in terms of medicine and not ethics" (Flynn 1991a: 182).

If the conflicts that emerged in committee discussions I observed, were picked up as something for decision-making, then, these conflicts were translated into a language that could make use of principles and regulations. Moreover, the decision-making was shifted to activities of the management department. Sometimes in the field research a language emerged that showed a struggling of how to talk about patients' concerns in a way that would portray the condition in all its little pieces of the situation best, but mostly a technical language was picked up. Terms like "case" which was very often used in the committees, but also "chances and risk" have "lost their anchor in the heart and the mind", borrowing Barbara Duden's vivid description (2002: 110).

I want to recall that the committees I observed were in a stage of establishment. Thus, the direction of their way of dealing with their issues of concern was not yet set. My interest was especially to see the ways of struggling with the brought up issues of concern in a multidisciplinary discussion, or to cite the field actors, how a debate would move when the "real conflicts" (Beck 2005) are at stake "to be tackled" (Alt 2006). At a later stage of committee development this investigation would have been more difficult, since then, the way of dealing with certain issues would have been more structured in a certain direction to keep the development running according to the forthcoming standards of how an ethics committee should work.

By doing and developing the steps of *Situational Analysis* (Adele Clarke 2005, see State of the Art, chapter two) for an understanding of the phenomenon of Hospital Ethics Committees, I could describe the historical background from different perspectives, identify silences and exclusions in the discourse as well as new questions which emerged from the data gained in the field. The observation of social phenomena in their "natural" setting, that is to say, sitting and watching behind closed doors of Hospital Ethics Committees, was an adequate way of bringing up data that could reveal "how practices at a certain place and at a certain time in a group develop" (Geertz 1990: 138).

Understanding "setting" in its double meaning, combined the following: First in its meaning of surrounding, and second, in its meaning of arena. In the research of three Hospital Ethics Committees, the importance of the surroundings was demonstrated by giving the case story of each committee in the surrounding of the hospital. The arenas of the committees' practices were then put into the foreground of the analysis. The double meaning of setting as a surrounding and arena was usable to sketch the field research not only as a field analysis, but also as a mode of presentation. By the unique capabilities of the field research, the subjects could be made audible and understandable as individuals and hereby; a counterbalance is given to the way of shaping societal actors by abstract notions that can deprive them of their essential human qualities.

Combining the findings of the three parts of my research, I resume the following: Communicative patterns in the observed Hospital Ethics Committees are embedded in a much broader discourse of (bio-) ethics, whose traces are disputable. Its contemporary rules of formation are gradually pervading the language of the actors in health care and limit the possibilities of thinking in terms of human relationships rather than rules.

The findings show that care is not a matter of natural practice for the daily clinical work as known in the tradition of Hippocratic ethic, but that the care ethos is rather at stake. Traditional care practices are replaced by a practice of administrative assignation. Like other institutions, hospitals are caught up with rationalisation procedures that can be easily measured in terms of outcomes, economic exchanges and accounting procedures. Caring is not understood as a relationship-based practice, but is turned into fractured care unities, delivered punctually by the interest of the institution and constrained by strict procedures.

A language of care in its most characteristic features and applications reminds people of an uncontrollable vulnerability, as well as its implications for dependency. It is much less disturbing when vulnerability remains private, and this in the sense of keeping it not only less socially expensive, but also out of sight and out of mind. Drawing on the language of management, efficiency and standardisation in the institution of the hospital, knowledge and skills of caring practices that cannot be predicted or controlled are "discounted".

There is a dilemma emerging: Exposing vulnerabilities in the language of care or keeping vulnerabilities and dependencies out of sight and mind in the language of "managed care". The language of care can hardly be translated into public, legal and accounting systems since these systems are designed to accommodate business transactions between strangers. Patients are neither clients nor strangers to physicians and nurses. The relationship is based on trust, truth and touch. Looking at the development of Hospital Ethics Committees in Germany, this is meant to be defended.

List of Abbreviations

AAB	American Association of Bioethics
ABA	American Breeder's Association
ADL	Activities of Daily Life
AEM	Academy for Ethics Medicine
ANA	American Nurses' Association
ASBH	American Society for Bioethics and Humanities
CEC	Clinical Ethics Consultation
CEC	Clinical Ethics Committee
CHA	Catholic Hospital Committee
CHO	Catholic Hospital Organization
DHHS	Department of Health and Human Services
DNR	Do Not Resuscitate
ED	Emergency Department
HEC	Hospital Ethics Committee
HEW	Department of Health, Education and Welfare
ICU	Intensive Care Unit
IEC	Institutional Ethics Committee
IRB	Institutional Review Board
JCAHO	The Joint Commission for the Accreditation of Health Care
LMED	Lower Mainland Emergency Department
MCO	Managed Care Organization
MD	Medical Doctor
MGH	Massachusetts General Hospital

MNA   Mini Nutritional Assessment

NEC   Nursing Ethics Committee

NICU   Neonatal Intensive Care Unit

OCC   Optimum Care Committee

RN   Registered Nurse

SBC   Society for Bioethics Consultation

SHHV   Society for Health and Human Values

ZfG   *Zentrum für Gesundheitsethik*

References

Agich, George J.; Youngner, Stuart J. (1991): For Experts Only? Access to Hospital Ethics Committees. *Hastings Center Report*, Sept.-Oct. 1991: 17–25.

Aiken, Linda H.; Clarke, Sean P.; Sloane, Douglas M. (2000): Hospital Restructuring: Does it adversely affect care and outcomes? *Journal of Nursing Administration*, 30 (10): 457–465.

Aiken, Linda H.; Clarke, Sean P.; Sloane, Douglas M. et al. (2001): Nurses' Reports On Hospital Care in Five Countries. *Health Affairs*, May / June 20 (3): 43–53.

Aikens, Charlotte A. (1916): *Studies in ethics for nurses*. Philadelphia.

Alexander, Shana (1962): They decide who lives, Who dies: Medical Miracle Puts a Moral Burden on a Small Community. *Life*, (9): 53.

American Academy of Paediatrics, Committee on Bioethics (2001): Institutional Ethics Committees. *Paediatrics*, 107 (1): 2005–2009.

American Hospital Association (1985): Ethics Committees double since '83. Survey. *Hospitals*, 39 (21): 60–64.

American Nurses' Association (ANA) (1940): A Tentative Code. *American Journal of Nursing*, 40 (9): 977–980.

American Nurses' Association (ANA) (1976): *Code for Nurses with Interpretative Statements*. Kansas City.

American Nurses' Association (ANA) (1985): *Code for Nurses with Interpretative Statements*. Kansas City.

American Nurses' Association (ANA) (1991): *Standards of Clinical Nursing Practice*. Missouri.

American Nurses' Association (ANA) (2001): *Code of Ethics for Nurses with Interpretative Statements*. Washington.

American Society for Bioethics and Humanities (ASBH) (1998): *Core Competencies for Health Care Ethics Consultation*. Glenview, IL.

Andre, Judith (2002): *Bioethics as Practice*. Dordrecht.

Annas, George J.; Grodin, Michael (1993): *The Nazi Doctors' Trial and the Nuremberg Code*. New York.

Anspach, Renee (1993): *Deciding who lives: Fateful choices in the intensive care nursery*. Berkeley.

Arndt, Marianne (1996): *Ethik denken: Maßstäbe zum Handeln in der Pflege*. Stuttgart.

Arney, William R.; Bergen, Bernard J. (1984): *Medicine and the Management of Living. Taming the Last Great Beast.* Chicago, London.

Aroskar, Mila (1984): Health Care Professionals and Ethical Relationships on IECs. In: Cranford, Ronald E.: Doudera, A. Edward (ed.): *Institutional Ethics Committees and Health Care Decision Making.* Michigan: 218–225.

Aroskar, Mila A.; Moldow, Gay D.; Good, Charles M. (2004): Nurses' Voices: Policy, Practice and Ethics. *Nursing Ethics,* 11 (3): 268–276.

Aulisio, Mark P.; Arnold, Robert M.; Youngner, Stuart J. (1999): An Ongoing Conversation: The Task Force Report and Bioethics Consultation. *The Journal of Clinical Ethics,* 10 (1): 3–4.

Bartels, Dianne (1988): Ethics Committees and Critical Care: Allies of Adversaries? *Perspectives in Critical Care,* 1: 83–90.

Bartels, Dianne; Youngner, Stuart; Levine, June (1994): Health Care Ethics Forum '94: Ethics Committees: Living up to your potential. *AACN Clinical Issues,* 5: 313–23.

Beauchamp, Tom; Childress, James F. (1983): *Principles of Biomedical Ethics,* 2nd edition, New York.

Becker, Howard S. (1958): Problems of Interface and Proof in Participant Observation. *American Sociological Review:* 652–660.

Bell, J.; Whiton, J.; Connelly S. (1998): *Final report: Evaluation of NEH implementation of section 491 of Public Health Service Act, mandating a program of protection for research subjects.*

Benjamin, Martin; Curtis, Joy (1986): *Ethics in nursing.* New York.

Benner, Patricia (1994 a): The Tradition and Skill of Interpretative Phenomenology in Studying Health, Illness, and Caring Practices. In: Benner, Patricia (1994) (ed.): *Interpretative Phenomenology. Embodiment, Caring, and Ethics in Health and Illness.* Thousand Oaks, CA.: 99–127.

Benner, Patricia (1994 b): Caring as a way of knowing and not knowing. In: Philips, Susan S.; Benner, Patricia: *The Crisis of Care. Affirming and Restoring Practices in the Helping Professions.* Washington: 42–62.

Benner, Patricia (1997): A Dialogue between virtue ethics and care ethics. *Theoretical Medicine,* 18: 47–61. The Netherlands.

Benner, Patricia (2000): The roles of embodiment, emotion and lifeworld for rationality and agency in nursing practice. *Nursing Philosophy,* 1: 5–19.

Benner, Patricia; Tanner, Christine A.; Chesla, Catherine A. (1996): *Expertise in nursing practice: Caring, clinical judgement, and ethics.* New York.

Benner, Patricia; Wrubel, Judith (1989): *The Primacy of Caring – Stress and Coping in Health and Illness.* Menlo Park.

Bequaert Holmes, Helen; Purdy, Laura M. (ed.) (1992): *Feminist Perspectives in Medical Ethics.* Bloomington, Indianapolis.

Bernal, Ellen W. (1992): The Nurse as Patient Advocate. *Hastings Center Report,* 22 (4): 18–23.

Biller-Andorno, Nikola (2001): *Gerechtigkeit und Fürsorge. Zur Möglichkeit einer integrativen Medizinethik.* Frankfurt am Main.

Bishop, Anne; Scudder, John R. (1987): Nursing ethics in an age of controversy. *Advances in Nursing Science*, 9 (3): 34–43.

Bishop, Anne; Scudder, John R. (1990): *The Practical, Moral, and Personal Sense of Nursing. A Phenomenological Philosophy of Practice*. New York.

Bjorklund, Pamela (2004): Invisibility, Moral Knowledge and Nursing Work in the Writings of Joan Liaschenko and Patricia Rodney. *Nursing Ethics*, 11 (2): 110–121.

Blank, Robert H.; Merrick, Janna C. (ed.) (2005): *End-of-Life Decision Making. A Cross-National Study.*

Bobbert, Monika (2002): *Patientenautonomie und Pflege. Begründung und Anwendung eines moralischen Rechts*. Frankfurt / New York.

Bosk, Charles L. (2001): Irony, Ethnography, and Informed Consent. In: Hoffmaster, Barry (ed.): *Bioethics in Social Context*. Philadelphia: 199–220.

Bosk, Charles L.; Frader, Joel (1998): Institutional Ethics Committees: Sociological Oxymeron, Empirical Black Box. In: DeVries, Raymond; Subedi, Janardan (ed.): *Bioethics and Society. Constructing the Ethical Enterprise*. New Jersey: 92–102.

Bourdieu, Pierre (1990): *The Logic of Practice*. California.

Braun, Kathrin (1999): Grenzen des Diskurses. Biomedizin, Bioethik und demokratischer Diskurs. In: Barben, Daniel; Abels, Gabriele (ed.): *Biotechnologie – Globalisierung – Demokratie. Politische Gestaltung transnationaler Technologieentwicklung*. Berlin: 409–429.

Braun, Kathrin (2000): *Menschenwürde und Biomedizin. Zum philosophischen Diskurs der Bioethik*. Frankfurt am Main.

Brennan, Troyen A. (1988): Ethics Committees and Decisions to Limit Care. The Experience at the Massachusetts General Hospital. *JAMA* 260 (6): 803–807.

Broberg, Gunnar; Roll-Hansen, Nils (ed.) (2005): *Eugenics in the Welfare State. Sterilisation Policy in Denmark, Sweden, Norway and Finland*. East Lansing.

Brody, Howard (2002): Narrative Ethics and Institutional Impact. In: Charon, Rita; Montello, Martha (ed.): *Stories Matter. The Role of Narrative Ethics*. New York: 149–153.

Bubeck, Diemut E. (1995): *Care, gender, and justice*. Oxford.

Brucker, Carola M. (1990): *Moralstrukturen. Grundlagen der Care-Ethik*. Weinheim.

Bruyn, Severyn T. (1963): The Methodology of Participant Observation. *Human Organisation:* 22.

Bundesministerium der Justiz (BMJ) (ed.) (2004): *Patientenautonomie am Lebensende – Ethische, rechtliche und medizinische Aspekte zur Bewertung von Patientenverfügungen, Bericht der Arbeitsgruppe "Patientenautonomie am Lebensende" vom 10. Juni 2004*. http://www.bmj.bund.de/media/archive/695.pdf

Buse, Gunhild (1993): *Macht – Moral – Weiblichkeit. Eine feministisch-theologische Auseinandersetzung mit Carol Gilligan und Frigga Haug*. Mainz.

Calhoun, Cheshire (1988): Justice, Care, Gender Bias. *Journal of Philosophy*, 85: 451–63.

Callahan, Daniel (1980): Contemporary Biomedical Ethics. *The New England Journal of Medicine*, 302: 1228–1233.

Callahan, Daniel (1984): Autonomy: A Moral Good, Not a Moral Obsession. *Hastings Center Report*, 14 (5): 40–42.

Caplan, Arthur L. (1987): Doing Ethics by Committees: Problems and Pitfalls. *The American Association for Laboratory Animal Science*: 45–47.

Caplan, Arthur L. (1989): Moral Experts and Moral Expertise. Do Either Exist? In: Hoffmaster, Barry; Freedman, Benjamin; Fraser, Gwen. Clifton (ed.): *Clinical Ethics. Theory and Practice*. New Jersey: 59–86.

Carse, Alisa L. (1991): The Voice of Care: Implications for Bioethical Education. *The Journal of Medicine and Philosophy*, 16: 5–28.

Carse, Alisa L; Lindemann Nelson, Hilde (1996): Rehabilitating Care. *Kennedy Institute of Ethics*, 6 (1): 19–35.

Castell, Robert (2001): From dangerousness to risk. In: Burchell, Graham; Gordon, Colin; Miller, Peter (ed.): *The Foucault Effect. Studies in Governmentality. With two Lectures by and an Interview with Michel Foucault*. Chicago.

Chambers, Tod (2000): Centering Bioethics. *Hastings Center Report*, 30 (1): 22–29.

Chambliss, Daniel F. (1996): *Beyond Caring. Hospitals, Nurses, and the Social Organization of Ethics*. Chicago.

Clarke, Adele E. (2005): *Situational Analysis. Grounded Theory after the Postmodern Turn*. Thousand Oaks.

Condon, Esther H. (1991): Nursing and the Caring Metaphor: Gender and Political Influences on an Ethics of Care. *Nursing Outlook*, 40 (1): 14–17.

Conradi, Elisabeth (2001): *Take Care. Grundlagen einer Ethik der Achtsamkeit*. Frankfurt, New York.

Conradi, Elisabeth (2003): Vom Besonderen zum Allgemeinen – Zuwendung in der Pflege als Ausgangspunkt einer Ethik. In: Behrendt, H.; Erichson, N.; Wiesemann, C. (ed.): *Pflege und Ethik. Leitfaden für Wissenschaft und Praxis*. Stuttgart: 30–46.

Cranford, Ronald E. (2002): *The History of Ethics Consultation in the United States: A Brief Review*. http:/clevelandclinic.org/bioethics/cec/plenary_cranford.htm 25.04.05, 12.55 h.

Cranford, Ronald E.; Doudera, A. Edward (1984): The Emergence of Institutional Ethics Committees. *Law, Medicine & Ethics*, 12 (1): 13–20.

Crigger, Bette-Jane (1995): Negotiating the Moral Order. Paradoxes of Ethics Consultation. *Kennedy Institute of Ethics Journal*, 5: 89–112.

Curtin, Leah L. (1979): The Nurse as Advocate: A Philosophical Foundation of Nursing. *Advances in Nursing Science*, 1 (3): 1–10.

Dallmann, Hans-Ulrich (2003): Fürsorge als Prinzip? Überlegungen zur Grundlegung einer Pflegeethik. *Zeitschrift für evangelische Ethik*, (47): 6–20.

David, Matthew; Sutton, Carole, D. (2004): *Social Research. The Basics*. London.

Davis, Anne J.; Aroskar, Mila A. (1983): *Ethical Dilemmas in Nursing Practice*. 2nd edition. London.

Davis, Anne J.; Aroskar, Mila A.; Liaschenko, Joan; Drought, Theresa S. (1997): *Ethical Dilemmas in Nursing Practice.* 4th edition. London.

Deitrich, G.; Belle-Haueisen, J., Mittelstaedt, G.v. (2003): Ist-Analyse der Ernährungssituation von mit PEG-Sonde versorgten älteren Menschen. Analysis of the Actual State of Nutrition of Elderly Patients Fed via PEG Tube. *Gesundheitswesen*, 65: 204–209.

De Moissac, Donna M.; Fay F. (1996): The Evolution of Caring within Bioethics: Provision for Relationship and context. *Nursing Ethics*, 3 (3): 191–201.

Department of Health and Human Services (1981): Rules and Regulations for Institutional Review Boards. *Federal Register*, 45 (16): 8375.

Department of Health and Human Services (1991): *Protection of Human Subjects.* Title 45 CFR § 46. June 18.

DeRenzo, Evan G.; Strass, Michelle (1997): A Feminist Model for Clinical Ethics Consultation: Increasing Attention to Context and Narrative. *HEC Forum*, 9 (3): 212–227.

Deutscher Bundestag (ed.) (2004): Zwischenbericht der Enquetekommission "Ethik und Recht der modernen Medizin" – Patientenverfügung. *Drucksache:* 15 / 3700 vom 13.09.2004. http://www.bundestag.de/parlament/kommissionen/ethik_med/berichte_stellg./04_09_13_zwischenbericht_patientenverfuegungen.pdf

Deutscher Evangelischer Krankenhausverband e. V, Katholischer Krankenhausverband Deutschlands e.V. (1997): *Ethik-Komitee im Krankenhaus.* Berlin / Freiburg.

Deutscher Evangelischer Krankenhausverband e. V, Katholischer Krankenhausverband Deutschlands e.V. (1999): *Ethik-Komitee im Krankenhaus. Erfahrungsberichte zur Einrichtung von Klinischen Ethik-Komitee.* Berlin / Freiburg.

DeVries, Raymond (2003): How Can We Help? From "Sociology in" to "Sociology of" Bioethics. *Journal of Law, Medicine & Ethics*, 32: 1–14.

DeVries, Raymond; Conrad, Peter (1998): Why Bioethics Needs Sociology. In: De Vries, Raymond; Subedi, Janardan (ed.): *Bioethics and Society. Constructing the Ethical Enterprise.* New Jersey: 233–257.

DeVries, Raymond; Forsberg, Carl P. (2002): Who Decides? A Look at Ethics Committee Membership. *HEC Forum*, 14 (3): 252–258.

Dodd, Sarah-Jane; Jansson, Bruce S.; Brown-Saltzman, Katherine et al. (2004): Expanding Nurses' Participation in Ethics: An Empirical Examination of Ethical Activism and Ethical Assertiveness. *Nursing Ethics*, 11 (1): 15–27.

Dörries, Andrea; Hespe-Jungesblut, Katharina (2007): Die Implementierung Klinischer Ethikberatung in Deutschland. Ergebnisse einer bundesweiten Umfrage bei Krankenhäusern. *Ethik in der Medizin*, 19 (2): 148–156.

Dreyfus, Hubert L.; Rabinow, Paul (1983): *Michel Foucault. Beyond Structuralism and Hermeneutics.* 2nd edition. Chicago.

Dryzek, John S. (2000): *Deliberative Democracy and Beyond. Liberals, Critics, Contestations.* Oxford.

Duden, Barbara (2002): *Die Gene im Kopf – der Fötus im Bauch. Historisches zum Frauenkörper.* Hannover.

Dunlop, Margaret J. (1994): Is a Science of Caring Possible? In: Benner, Patricia (1994) (ed.): *Interpretative Phenomenology. Embodiment, Caring, and Ethics in Health and Illness.* Thousand Oaks, CA.: 27–42.

Düwell, Markus; Steigleder, Klaus (ed.) (2003): *Bioethik. Eine Einführung.* Frankfurt am Main.

Dzur, Albert (2002): Democratizing the Hospital: Deliberative-Democratic Bioethics. *Journal of Health Politics and Law,* Vol. 27 (2): 177–211.

Edwards, Barbara J.; Haddad, Amy M. (1988): Establishing a Nursing Bioethics Committee. *JONA,* 18 (3): 30–33.

Engelhardt, Tristram H., Jr. (1986): *The foundations of bioethics.* New York.

Engelhardt, Volker von Loewenich; Simon, Alfred (ed.) (2000): *Die Heilberufe auf der Suche nach ihrer Identität. Jahrestagung der Akademie für Ethik in der Medizin e.V.* Hamburg.

Erlen, Judith A. (1993): Empowering Nurses through Nursing Ethics Committees. *Orthopaedic Nursing,* 12 (2): 69–72.

Erlen, Judith A. (1997): Are Nursing Ethics Committees necessary? *HEC Forum,* 9 (1): 55–67.

Evans, John H. (2000): A Sociological Account of the Growth of Principlism. *Hastings Center Report,* September – October: 31–38.

Faden, R.R.; Beauchamp, J. (1986): *A History and Theory of Informed Consent.* New York.

Finkenbine, Ryan; Gramelspacher, Gregory (1991): Physicians' attitudes toward Hospital Ethics Committees. *Indiana Medicine,* November: 804–807.

Fischer, Michael (2003): Geld und Moral im Krankenhaus. Auf dem Weg zu einer Ethikkultur. In: Heller, Andreas; Krobath, Thomas (ed.): *Organisationsethik. Organisationsentwicklung in Kirchen, Caritas und Diakonie.* Freiburg im Breisgau: 419–428.

Fisher, Berenice; Tronto, Joan (1990): Toward a feminist theory of care. In: Abel, Emily; Nelson, Margaret (ed.): *Circles of Care: Work and Identity in Women's Life.* Albany, New York: 36–54.

Fleming, Cornelia M. (1997): The Establishment and Development of Nursing Ethics Committees. *HEC Forum,* (1): 7–19.

Fletcher, John C.; Siegler, Mark (1996): What are the goals of ethics consultation? A consensus statement. *Journal of Clinical Ethics,* 7 (2): 122–26.

Flick, Uwe (1996): *Qualitative Forschung. Theorie, Methoden, Anwendung in Psychologie und Sozialwissenschaften.* Reinbek bei Hamburg.

Flynn, Patricia (1991 a): *Moral ordering and the social construction of bioethics. Unpublished dissertation.* San Francisco.

Flynn, Patricia (1991 b): The Disciplinary Emergence of Bioethics and Bioethics Committees: Moral Ordering and its Legitimation. *Sociological Focus,* 24 (2): 145–156.

Fost, Norman; Cranford, Ronald E. (1985): Hospital Ethics Committees. Administrative Aspects. *JAMA,* 253 (18): 2687–2692.

Foucault, Michel (1974): *Die Ordnung der Dinge.* Frankfurt am Main.

Foucault, Michel (1986): *Die Sorge um sich. Sexualität und Wahrheit.* Bd. 3. Frankfurt am Main.

Foucault, Michel (1988): Technologies of the Self. In: Martin, L; Gutman, H.; Hutton, P. (ed.): *Technologies of the Self. A Seminar with Michel Foucault.* Amherst: 73–86.

Foucault, Michel (1991): Governmentality. In: Burchell, Graham; Gordon, Collin; Miller, Peter (ed.): *The Foucault Effect. Studies in Governmentality.* Chicago.

Foucault, Michel (1991): Questions of Method. Burchell, C.; Gordon, C.; Miller, P. (ed.): *The Foucault Effect: Studies in Governmentality.* Chicago: 73–86.

Fowler, Marsha (1997): Nursing's Ethics. In: Davis, Anne J.; Aroskar, Mila A.; Liaschenko, Joan; Drought, Theresa S.: *Ethical Dilemmas in Nursing Practice.* 4th edition. London: 17–34.

Fox, Renee C. (1974): Ethical and Existential Developments in Contemporaneous American Medicine: Their Implications for Culture and Society. *Health and Society,* Fall: 445–481.

Fox, Renee C. (1979): *Essays in Medical Sociology. Journeys in into the field.* New York.

Fox, Renee C. (1989): *The Sociology of Medicine. A participant observer's view.* New Jersey.

Fox, Renee C. (1990): The Evolution of American Bioethics: A Sociological Perspective. In: Weisz (ed.): *Social Science Perspectives on Medical Ethics.* Pennsylvania: 201–217

Fox, Renee C. (1996): More than Bioethics. *Hastings Center Report,* November–December: 5–7.

Fox, Renee C.; Swazey, Judith P. (1974): *The courage to fail: A social view of organ transplantation and dialysis.* Chicago.

Fox, Renee C.; Swazey, Judith P. (1984): Medical Morality is Not Bioethics – Medical Ethics in China and the United States. *Perspectives in Biology and Medicine,* 27 (3): 337–360.

Frader, Joel E. (1992): Political and interpersonal aspects of ethics consultation. *Theoretical Medicine,* (13): 31–44.

Frenkel, David A. (2003): The Role of the Ethics Committee in Hospital Practice. In: *Medicine and Law,* 22: 227–633.

Friedrichs, Jürgen (1985): *Methoden empirischer Sozialforschung.* Opladen.

Friesacher, Heiner (2004): Foucaults Konzept der Gouvernementalität als Analyseinstrument für die Pflegewissenschaft. *Pflege,* (17): 364–374.

Fry, Sarah T. (1988): The ethic of caring. Can it survive in nursing? *Editorial Nursing Outlook,* 36 (1): 48.

Fry, Sarah T. (1989): Toward a theory of nursing ethics. *Advances in Nursing Science,* 11 (4): 9–22.

Fry, Sarah T. (1992): The Role of Caring in a Theory of Nursing Ethics. In: Bequaert Holmes, Helen; Purdy, Laura M. (ed.): *Feminist Perspectives in Medical Ethics*. Bloomington, Indianapolis: 93–106.

Fry, Sarah T. (1994): Ethics in Nursing Practice. *A Guide to Ethical Decision Making*. Genf.

Fry, Sarah T.; Harvey, R.M.; Hurley, A.C.; Fowley, B.J. (2002): Development of a model of moral distress in military. *Nursing Ethics*, 9 (4): 373–387.

Gadamer, H.G. (1990): *Wahrheit und Methode*. Gesammelte Werke. Bd. 1. Tübingen.

Gadow, Sally (1980): "Existential Advocacy: Philosophical Foundation of Nursing". In: Gadow, Sally; Spicker, Stuart F. (ed.): *Nursing Images and Ideals. Opening Dialogue with the Humanities*. New York: 79–101.

Gadow, Sally (1984): Touch and Technology: Two Paradigms of Patient Care. *Journal of Religion and Health*, 23 (1): 63–69.

Gadow, Sally (1985): Nurse and Patient: The Caring Relationship. In: Bishop, Anne H.; Scudder, John R. (ed.): *Caring, Curing, Coping. Nurse, Physician, Patient, Relationships*. Birmingham: 31–43.

Geertz, Clifford (1973): *The Interpretation of Cultures*. New York.

Geertz, Clifford (1990): *Die künstlichen Wilden*. München.

Giese, Constanze; Koch, Christian; Siewert, Dietmar (2006): Sterbehilfe – kein Thema für die Pflege? *Dr. med. Mabuse*, Nr. 164, Nov. / Dez.: 43–46.

Gillen, Erny (1999): Frag nur – ethische Reflexionen zu den Fragestellungen im Klinischen Ethik-Komitee. In: Deutscher Evangelischer Krankenhausverband e.V. / Katholischer Krankenhausverband Deutschlands e.V. (ed.) (1999): *Ethikkomitee im Krankenhaus. Erfahrungsberichte zur Einrichtung von Klinischen Ethik-Komitees:* 10–15.

Gilligan, Carol (1982): *In a different voice. Psychological Theory and Women's Development*. Massachusetts.

Gladwin, Mary E. (1937): *Ethics: A textbook for nurses*. Philadelphia.

Glaser, Barney G.; Strauss, Anselm L. (1967): *The Discovery of Grounded Theory. Strategies for Qualitative Research*. New York.

Glaser, Barney G.; Strauss, Anselm L. (1974): *Interaktion mit Sterbenden. Beobachtungen für Ärzte, Schwestern, Seelsorger und Angehörige*. Übs.: Bischoff-Elten, Gisela. Göttingen.

Gordon, Suzanne (1997): What nurses stand for? *Atlantic Monthly*, 279 (2): 81–88.

Gorovitz, Samuel et al. (ed.) (1976): *Moral Problems in Medicine*. New Jersey.

Grace, Pamela J. (2001): Professional advocacy: Widening the Scope of Accountability. *Nursing Philosophy*, 2: 151–162.

Graeve, Stefanie (2007): Im Schatten des Homo oeconomicus. Subjektmodelle "am Lebensende" zwischen Einwilligungs(un)fähigkeit und Ökonomisierung. In: Krasmann, Susanne; Volkmer, Michael (ed.): *Michel Foucaults "Geschichte der Gouvernementalität" in den Sozialwissenschaften. Internationale Beiträge*. Bielefeld: 267–286.

Gramelspacher, Gregory P.; Howell, Joel D.; Young, Mark J. (1986): Perceptions of Ethical Problems by Nurses and Doctors. *Arch Intern Med,* 146: 577–578.

Gray, Bradford H. (1975): An Assessment of Institutional Review Committees in Human Experimentation. *Medical Care,* 13 (1975): 318–328.

Grekul, Jana; Krahn, Harvey; Odynak, Dave (2004): Sterilizing the "Feeble-minded": Eugenics in Alberta, Canada, 1929–1972. *Journal of Historical Sociology,* 17 (4): 358–384.

Griener, Glenn G.; Storch, Janet L. (1992): "Hospital Ethics Committees: Problems in Evaluation". *Hospital Ethics Committee Forum,* 4: 5–18.

Griener, Glenn G.; Storch, Janet L. (1994): "Educational Needs of Hospital Ethics Committees". *Cambridge Quarterly of Healthcare Ethics,* 3: 467–477.

Grob, Gerald N. (1991): Foreword. In: Reilly, Philip R.: *The Surgical Solution. A History of Involuntary Sterilization in the United States.* Baltimore: IX–XI.

Großklaus-Seidel, Marion (2002): *Ethik im Pflegealltag. Wie Pflegende ihr Handeln reflektieren und begründen können.* Stuttgart.

Haraway, Donna (1985): A manifesto for Cyborgs: Science, Technology, and Social Feminism in the 1980s. *Social Review,* 80: 65–105.

Haraway, Donna (1988): Situated Knowledges: The Science Question in Feminism and the Privilege of Partial Perspective. *Feminist Studies,* 14 (3): 575–599.

Hardingham, Lorraine B. (2004): Integrity and moral residue: nurses as participants in a moral community. *Nursing Philosophy,* 5: 127–134.

Hayes, G.J.; Hayes, S.C.; Dykstra, T. (1995): A survey of university institutional review boards: Characteristics, policies and procedures. *IRB,* 17 (3): 1–6.

Hedgecoe, Adam M. (2004): Critical Bioethics: Beyond the Social Science Critique of Applied Ethics. *Bioethics,* 18 (2): 121–143.

Held, Virginia (1993): *Feminist Morality. Transforming Culture, Society, and Politics.* Chicago, London.

Hoffmann, Diane E. (1993): Evaluating Ethics Committees: A View from the Outside. *The Milbank Quarterly,* 71 (4): 677–701.

Hoffmann, Diane E.; Tarzian, Anne J.; O'Neil, J. Anne (2000): Are ethics committees members competent to consult? *Journal of Law, Medicine, and Ethics,* 28 (1): 30–40.

Hoffmaster, Barry (1992): Can Ethnography Save the Life of Medical Ethics? *Social Science Medicine,* 35 (12): 1421–1431.

Hoffmaster, Barry (ed.) (2001): *Bioethics in Social Context.* Philadelphia.

Holly, Cheryl Malahan (1986): *Staff Nurses' Participation in Ethical Decision Making: A descriptive Study of selected Situational Variables.* Unpublished dissertation. Columbia.

Holmes, Dave; Gestaldo, Denise (2002): Nursing as a means of governmentality. *Journal of Advanced Nursing,* 18: 557–565.

Holmes, Helen B.; Purdy, Laura M. (1992): *Feminist Perspectives in Medical Ethics.* Bloomington.

Igoe, Sharon E.; Goncalves, Susan A. (1997): Nursing Ethics Committees and Policy Development. *HEC Forum,* 9 (1): 20–26.

Illich, Ivan (1981): *Die Nemesis der Medizin*. München.

Illich, Ivan; Caley, David (2007): *In den Flüssen nördlich der Zukunft*. München.

Jaggar, Alison (1995): Caring as a Feminist Practice of Moral Reason. In: Held, Virginia (ed.): *Justice and Care. Essential Readings in Feminist Ethics*. Boulder: 179–202.

Jameton, Andrew (1984): *Nursing Practice. The ethical issues*. New Jersey.

Johnstone, Megan-Jane (1994): *Bioethics. A nursing perspective*. Sydney.

Joint Commission on the Accreditation of Healthcare Organizations (1992): *Accreditation Manual for Hospitals:* 103–105.

Jonsen, A. R. (1998): *The Birth of Bioethics*. New York, Oxford.

Jonsen, A. R.; Siegler, M.; Winslade, W. (1998): *Clinical Ethics: A Practical Approach to Ethical Decisions in Clinical Medicine*. 4ᵗʰ Edition, New York.

Kalchbrenner, Joan; Kelly, Margaret J.; McCarthy, Donald G. (1983): Ethics Committees and Ethicists in Catholic Hospitals. *Hospital Progress:* 47–51.

Käppeli, Silvia (1988): Moralisches Handeln und berufliche Unabhängigkeit in der Krankenpflege. *Pflege*, (1): 20–27.

Käppeli, Silvia (2001): Mit-Leiden – eine vergessene Tradition in der Pflege? *Pflege*, (5): 293–306.

Käppeli, Silvia (2004): *Vom Glaubenswerk zur Pflegewissenschaft. Geschichte des Mit-Leidens in der christlichen, jüdischen und freiberuflichen Krankenpflege*. Bern.

Katz-Rothman, Barbara (2001): *The book of life: a personal and ethical guide to race, normality, and the implications of the human genome project*. Boston, Massachusetts.

Katz, Alfred H.; Proctor, D. M. (1969): Social-Psychological Characteristics of Patients Receiving Haemodialysis in Treatment for Chronic Renal Failure. *Public Health Service, Kidney Disease Control Program*.

Kaufmann, Sharon (2005): *... And a Time to Die. How American Hospitals Shape the End of Life*. New York.

Keenan, Carol (1983): Ethics Committees: trend for troubling times. *The Hospital Medical Staff,* June: 2–8

Keffer, Jan M. (1997): Why Nursing Ethics Committees? *HEC Forum*, 9 (1): 50–54.

Kettner, Matthias (2005): Ethik-Komitees. Ihre Organisationsformen und ihr moralischer Anspruch. *Erwägen Wissen Ethik (EWE)*, 16 (1): 3–16.

Kettner, Matthias; May, Arnd (2002): Ethik-Komitees in Kliniken – Bestandsaufnahme und Zukunftsperspektiven. *Ethik in der Medizin*, 14 (4): 295–297.

Kittay, Eva F. (1999): *Love's Labor: Essays on Women, Equality, and Dependency*. New York.

Kittay, Eva F. (2004): Behinderung und das Konzept der Care-Ethik. In: Graumann, Sigrid; Grüber, Kathrin; Nicklas-Faust, Jeanne et. al. (ed.): *Ethik und Behinderung. Ein Perspektivwechsel*. Frankfurt am Main.

Kleinman, Arthur; Fox, Renee C.; Brandt, Allan M. (1999): *Bioethics and Beyond*. Daedalus.

Klockenbusch, W. (1986): *Die Betreuung unheilbar Kranker und Sterbender. Psychische Belastungen des Krankenpflegepersonals.* Melsungen.

Kohlberg, Lawrence (1981): *The Philosophy of Moral Development. Moral Stages and the Idea of Justice. Essays on Moral Development.* San Francisco.

Kohlen, Helen (2006): *Troubled Voices of Care. Formen der Regulierung durch Krankenhaus-Ethikkomitees.* Presentation at Centre Marc Bloch; Conference Internationale: Ethique du Care, Politiques du Care. Unpublished paper. Berlin.

Kohlen, Helen (2007): Patientenautonomie aus der Sicht der Pflege und Perspektiven einer Care-Ethik. In: Charbonnier, Ralph; Dörner, Klaus; Steffen, Simon (ed.): *Patientenwille und medizinische Indikation.* Stuttgart.

Kohnke, Mary F. (1980): The nurse as Advocate. *American Journal of Nursing,* November: 2030–2040.

Körtner, Ulrich J.H. (2004): *Grundkurs Pflegeethik.* Wien.

Kuhse, Helga (1995): Clinical Ethics and Nursing: "Yes" to Caring, but "No" to a Female Ethics of Care. *Bioethics,* Volume 9, Number ¾: 207–219.

Lamnek, Siegfried (1995): *Qualitative Sozialforschung.* 3.Auflage. Band 2. Methoden und Techniken. Weinheim.

Lanoix, Monique (2006): The Problem of High-Maintenance Bodies or the Politics of Care. In: Beaulieu, Alain; Gabbard, David (ed.): *Michel Foucault and Power Today. International Multidisciplinary Studies in the History of the Present.* Lanham, Boulder, New York, Toronto, Oxford: 93–104.

La Puma, John; Stocking, Carol B.; Darling, Cheryl M.; Siegler, M. (1992): Community Hospital Ethics Consultation: Evaluation and Comparison with a University Hospital Service. *The American Journal of Medicine,* 92: 346–351.

Langer, Elionor (1966): Human Experimentation: New York Verdict Affirms Patient's Right. *Science,* 151: 663–666.

Lay, Reinhard (2004): *Ethik in der Pflege. Ein Lehrbuch für die Aus-, Fort- und Weiterbildung.* Hannover.

Lessing, Doris (1972): *The Golden Notebook.* 2nd edition, London.

Levine, Carol (1984): Questions and (some very tentative) answers about hospital ethics committees. *Hastings Center Report,* 14 (3): 9–12.

Levine, Robert J. (1986): *Ethics and Regulation of Clinical Research.* 2nd editon. Baltimore.

Liaschenko, Joan (1993a): *Faithful to the good: Morality and philosophy in nursing practice.* Unpublished doctoral dissertation. University of California, San Francisco.

Liaschenko, Joan (1993b): Feminist ethics and cultural ethos: Revisiting a nursing debate. *Advances in Nursing Science,* 1993, 15 (4): 71–81.

Liaschenko, Joan (1995a): Ethics in the work of acting for patients. *Advances in Nursing Science,* 18 (2): 1–12.

Liaschenko, Joan (1995b): Artificial Personhood: Nursing Ethics in a Medical World. *Nursing Ethics,* 2 (3): 185–196.

Liaschenko, Joan (1997): Knowing the patient? In: Thorne, Sally E.; Hayes, Virginia E. (ed.): *Nursing praxis: Knowledge and action.* Thousand Oaks: 23–38.

Liaschenko, Joan (2001): Thoughts on nursing work. *Bioethics Examiner*, 5 (2): 2–6.

Liaschenko, Joan; Fisher, Anastasia; (1999): Theorizing the Knowledge that Nurses use in the Conduct of their Work. Scholarly Inquiry for Nursing Practice: *An International Journal*, 13 (1): 29–41.

Liaschenko, Joan; Peter, Elisabeth (2003): Whose morality is it anyway? Thoughts on the work of Margaret Urban Walker. *Nursing Philosophy*, 4: 259–262.

Lindemann, Hilde (2006): *An Invitation to Feminist Ethics.* New York.

Lipp, Volker (2005): *Patientenautonomie und Lebensschutz. Zur Diskussion um eine gesetzliche Regelung der "Sterbehilfe".* Göttingen.

Lo, Bernard (1987): "Behind close doors: Promises and Pitfalls of an Ethics Committee". *New England Journal of Medicine*, 317 (1): 46–49.

Lo, Bernard (2003): Answers and Questions About Ethics Consultation. *JAMA*, September 3, 290 (9): 1208–1210.

Logan, Winnifred; Roper, Nancy; Tierney, Allison J. (2002): *Das Roper-Logan-Tierney-Modell. Basierend auf Lebensaktivitäten (LA).* Bern 2002.

Macklin, Ruth (1987): *Mortal choices.* New York.

Macklin, Ruth (1988): The Inner Workings of an Ethics Committee: Latest Battle over Jehovah's Witnesses. *The Hastings Center Report*, 18 (1): 15–20.

Macklin, Ruth; Robin B. Kupfer (1988): *Hospital Ethics Committees: Manual for a training program.* New York: Albert Einstein College of Medicine.

Maslow, Abraham L. (1959): *New Knowledge in Human Values.* New York.

May, Arndt T. (2004): Ethische Entscheidungsfindung in der klinischen Praxis. Die Rolle klinischer Ethikkomitees. *Ethik in der Medizin*, (16): 242–252.

Mayntz, Renate; Holm, Kurt; Hübner, Peter (1978): *Einführung in die Methoden der empirischen Soziologie.* 5. Auflage. Opladen.

Mayring, Philipp (2002): *Einführung in die qualitative Sozialforschung.* Weinheim, Basel.

Mayring, Philipp (2003): *Qualitative Inhaltsanalyse. Grundlagen und Techniken.* Weinheim, Basel.

McBurney, Cate (2001): Ethics Committees and Social Change. Plus ca change? In: Hoffmaster, Barry (ed.): *Bioethics in Social Context.* Philadelphia: 180–199.

McCall, George J. (ed.) (1969): *Issues in Participant Observation: A Text and Reader.* Chicago.

McCormick, Richard A. (1984): Ethics committees: promise or peril? *Law, Medicine & Health Care*, 12 (4): 150–155.

McDaniel, Charlotte (1998): Hospital Ethics Committees and Nurses' Participation. *JONA*, 28 (9): 47–51.

Medizinischer Dienst der Spitzenverbände der Krankenkassen e.V. (MDS) (ed.) (2003): *Ernährung und Flüssigkeitsversorgung älterer Menschen. Abschlussbericht.* Essen.

Meuser, Michael; Nagel, Ulrike (1991): Experteninterviews – vielfach erprobt, wenig bedacht. In: Garz, Detlef; Kraimer, Klaus (ed.): *Qualitative empirische Sozialforschung. Konzepte, Methoden, Analysen.* Opladen: 441–471.

Meuser, Michael; Nagel, Ulrike (2003): Das Experteninterview – Wissenssoziologische Voraussetzungen und methodische Durchführung. In: Friebertshäuser, Barbara; Prengel, Annedore (ed.): *Handbuch Qualitative Forschungsmethoden in der Erziehungswissenschaft.* Weinheim: 481–491.

Miles, Steven (1987): Futile feeding at the end of life: Family virtues and treatment decisions. *Theoretical Medicine,* 8: 293–302.

Minogue, Brendan (1996): *Bioethics. A Committee Approach.* Boston, London, Singapore.

Mitchell, Gail J. (2001): Policy, procedure and routine: Matters of moral influence. *Nursing Science Quarterly,* 14 (2): 109–114.

Moreno, Jonathan D. (1995): *Deciding together. Bioethics and Moral Consensus.* New York, Oxford.

Morse, Janice M. (1990): Concepts of caring and caring as a concept. *Advanced Nursing Science,* 13 (1): 1–14.

Müller, Elke (2001): *Leitbilder in der Pflege. Eine Untersuchung individueller Pflegeauffassungen als Beitrag zu ihrer Präzisierung.* Bern.

Murphy, Patricia (1989): The Role of the Nurse on Hospital Ethics Committees. *Nursing Clinics of North America,* 24 (2): 551–555.

Muyskens, James L. (1982): *Moral problems in nursing: A philosophical investigation.* Totowa, New Jersey.

Nagl-Docekal, Herta; Pauer-Studer, Herlinde (ed.) (1993): *Jenseits der Geschlechtermoral.* Frankfurt am Main.

Neitzke, Gerald (2002): Ethische Konflikte im Stationsalltag. *Planetarium,* (42): 9–10.

Nelson, Hilde L. (1992): Against Caring. *Journal of Clinical Ethics,* (3): 8–20.

Nelson, James L. (2000): Moral Teachings from Unexpected Quarters. Lessons for Bioethics from the Social Sciences and Managed Care. *Hastings Center Report,* January – February: 12–17.

Neveloff Dubler, Nancy; Nimmons, David (1992): *Ethics on Call. A Medical Ethicist Shows How to Take Charge of Life-and-Death Choices.* New York.

New York State Task Force on Life and the Law (1986): *Do not resuscitate orders. The proposed legislation and report of the New York State Task Force on Life and the Law.* New York.

Noddings, Nel (1984): Caring. *A Feminine Approach to Ethics and Morals Education.* Berkeley, California.

Nussbaum, Martha C. (1999): *Gerechtigkeit oder das gute Leben.* Frankfurt am Main 1999.

Oddi, Lorys F.; Cassidy, Virginia R. (1990): Participation and Perception of Nurse Members in the Hospital Ethics Committee. *Western Journal of Nursing Research,* 12 (3): 307–317.

Olbrich, Christa (1999): *Pflegekompetenz.* Bern, Göttingen, Toronto, Seattle.

Pellegrino, Edmund D. (1985): The caring ethic: The relation of physician to patient. In: Bishop, Anne H.; Scudder, John R., Jr. (ed.): *Caring, curing, coping. Nurse, physician, patient relationships.* Birmingham, Alabama.

Pellegrino, Edmund D. (1993): The Metamorphis of Medical Ethics. A 30-Year Retrospective. *JAMA*, 269 (9): 1158–1162.

Pellegrino, Edmund D.; Thomasma, David C. (1988): *For the patient's good*. New York: Oxford University Press.

Perini, Corina; Stauffer, Yvonne; Grunder, Margrit et al. (2006): Die Bedeutung von Caring aus der Sicht von Patienten mit chronischen Wunden bei Peripher Arteriellen Verschlusskrankheiten. *Pflege*, Heft 19: 345–355.

Pfau-Effinger, Birgit; Geissler, Birgit (ed.) (2005): *Care and Social Integration in European Societies*. Bristol.

Philips, Susan S.; Benner, Patricia (1994): *The Crisis of Care. Affirming and Restoring Practices in the Helping Professions*. Washington.

Piaget, Jean (1932): *The Moral Judgement of the Child*. New York.

Pinch, Winifried J. Ellenchild (2002): *When the Bough Breaks. Parental Perceptions of Ethical Decision-Making in NICU*. Lanham, New York, Oxford.

President's Commission for the Study of Ethical Problems in Medicine and Biomedical and Behavioural Research (1983): *Deciding to Forego Life-Sustaining Treatment*. Washington D.C.

Purtilo, Ruth; Haddad, Amy (2002): *Health Professional and Patient Interaction*. 6th edition. Philadelphia, London.

Rabe, Marianne (2000): Dienst am Nächsten oder professionelle Fürsorge. Werte für die Krankenpflege. *Berliner Medizinethische Schriften. Beiträge zu ethischen und rechtlichen Fragen der Medizin*, Heft 37. Dortmund.

Randal, Judith (1983): Are Ethics Committees Alive and Well? *The Hastings Center Report*, 13 (6): 10–12.

Rafeal, Adeline R. Falk (1996): Power and Caring: A dialectic in Nursing. *Advanced Nursing Science*, 19 (1): 3–17.

Rawls, John (1971): A theory of justice. Cambridge, MA.

Redman, Barbara K. (1996): Responsibility of Healthcare Ethics Committees towards Nurses. *HEC Forum*, 8 (1): 52–60.

Rehbock, Theda (2002): Autonomie – Fürsorge – Paternalismus. Zur Kritik (medizin-) ethischer Grundbegriffe. *Ethik in der Medizin*, 14 (3): 131–150.

Reilly, Philip R. (1991): *The Surgical Solution. A History of Involuntary Sterilization in the United States*. Baltimore.

Reiser, Joel; Dyck, Arthur J.; Curran, William J. (ed.) (1977): *Ethics in Medicine. Historical Perspectives and Contemporary Concerns*. Cambridge, London.

Remmers, Hartmut (2000): *Pflegerisches Handeln. Wissenschafts- und Ethikdiskurse zur Konturierung der Pflegewissenschaft*. Bern, Göttingen, Toronto, Seattle.

Remmers, Hartmut (2003): *Patientenautonomie aus pflegeethischer Perspektive*. Unveröffentlichtes Vortragsmanuskript. Universität Osnabrück.

Reverby, Susan (1987): *Ordered to Care. The Dilemma of American Nursing*. Cambridge.

Robb, Isabel H. (1976): The spirit of the associated alumnae. In: Flanagan, L. (ed.): *One strong voice. The story of the ANA*. Kansas City.

Robertson, John A. (1984): Ethics Committees in Hospitals: Alternative Structures and Responsibilities. *Connecticut Medicine*, 48 (7): 441–444.

Rodney, Patricia A. (1997): *Towards connectedness and trust: Nurses' enactment of their moral agency within an organizational context*. Unpublished doctoral dissertation. University of British Columbia, Vancouver, Canada.

Rodney, Patricia A. (2005): Power, Politics, and Practice: Towards a Better Moral Climate for Health Care Delivery. *The 9th International Philosophy of Nursing Conference. Book of abstracts*. University of Leeds.

Rodney, Patricia A.; Varcoe, Colleen (2001): Toward ethical inquiry in the economic evaluation of nursing practice. *Canadian Journal of Nursing Research*, 33 (1): 35–37.

Rogers, Carl R. (1989): *On Becoming a Person. A Therapist's View of Psychotherapy*. Boston.

Rosner, Fred (1985): Hospital Medical Ethics Committees: A Review of their Development. *JAMA*, 253 (18): 2693–7.

Ross, Judith W. (1986): *Handbook for Hospital Ethics Committees. Practical suggestions for ethics committee members to plan, develop, and evaluate their roles and responsibilities*. Chicago.

Rothman, David J. (2003): *Strangers at the Bedside: A History of How Law and Bioethics Transformed Medical Decision Making*. New York.

Rubin, Susan; Zoloth-Dorfman, Laurie (1996): She Said / He Said: Ethics Consultation and the Gendered Discourse. *The Journal of Clinical Ethics*, 7 (4): 321–332.

Ruddick, Sara (1989): *Maternal Thinking. Toward a Politics of Peace*. New York.

Rues, Lawrence A. (1987): Starting an Institutional Ethics Committee: One Physician's Experience. Exploring the structure, function and scope of ethics committees. *Healthcare Executive*, 2 (4): 34–38.

Rushton, Cynda; Youngner, Stuart J.; Skeel, Joy (2003): Models for Ethics Consultation. Individual, Team, or Committee? In: Aulisio, Mark P.; Arnold, Robert M.; Youngner, Stuart J. (ed.): *Ethics Consultation. From Theory to Practice*. Baltimore.

Samerski, Silja (2002): *Die verrechnete Hoffnung. Von der selbstbestimmten Entscheidung durch genetische Beratung*. Münster.

Sarvis, Betty; Rodman, Hyman, (1974): *The Abortion Controversy*. Columbia.

Scheirton, Linda Sue (1990): *The Relationship between Ethics Committees Success and the Training and Status of the Chairperson in University Teaching Hospitals*. Unpublished dissertation. University of Austin, Texas.

Schmidt, Kurt W. (2001): Models of Ethics Consultation: The "Frankfurter Model". *HEC Forum*, 13 (3): 281–293.

Schneider, Ulrike (1980): *Sozialwissenschaftliche Methodenkrise und Handlungsforschung. Methodische Grundlagen der Kritischen Psychologie 2*. Frankfurt am Main.

Schnepp, Wilfried (1996): Pflegekundige Sorge. Deutsche Gesellschaft für Pflegewissenschaft e.V. (ed.): *Pflege und Gesellschaft*. Duisburg.

Schües, Christina (2000): Leben als Geborene – Handeln in Beziehung. Feministische Ethik im Anschluss an Arendts Gedanken der Natalität. In: Conradi, Elisabeth; Plonz, Sabine (ed.): *Tätiges Leben. Pluralität und Arbeit im politischen Denken Hannah Arendts*. Bochum: 67–93.

Schwartz, Morris S.; Schwartz, Charlotte G. (1955): Problems in Participant Observation. *American Journal of Sociology:* 343–353.

Schwerdt, Ruth (2002): *Ethisch-moralische Kompetenzentwicklung als Indikator für Professionalisierung. Das Modellprojekt "Implementierung ethischen Denkens in den beruflichen Alltag Pflegender".* Regensburg.

Sherwin, Susan (1992): *No longer patient: Feminist ethics and health care.* Philadelphia.

Sichel, Betty A. (1992): Ethics of Caring and the Institutional Ethics Committee. In: Bequaert Holmes, Helen; Purdy, Laura M. (ed.): *Feminist Perspectives in Medical Ethics.* Bloomington, Indianapolis: 113–123.

Simms, Mary (1989): Social Research and the Rationalization of Care. In: Gubrium, Jaber F.; Silverman, David (ed.): *The Politics of Field Research. Sociology beyond Enlightenment.* London: 173–196.

Simon, Alfred (2000): Klinische Ethikberatung in Deutschland. Erfahrungen aus dem Krankenhaus Neu-Mariahilf in Göttingen. *Berliner Medizinethische Schriften,* 36. Dortmund.

Simon, Alfred; Gillen, Erny (2000): Klinische Ethik-Komitees in Deutschland. Feigenblatt oder praktische Hilfestellung in Konfliktsituationen? In: Engelhardt, Volker von Loewenich; Simon, Alfred (ed.) (2000): *Die Heilberufe auf der Suche nach ihrer Identität. Jahrestagung der Akademie für Ethik in der Medizin e.V.* Hamburg: 151–157.

Slowther, Anne-Marie; Hope, Tony (2000): Clinical ethics committees: They can change clinical practice but need evaluation. *British Medical Journal 321,* September: 649–650.

Smith, Dorothy E. (1990): *The Conceptual Practices of Power. A Feminist Sociology of Knowledge.* Boston.

Smith, Dorothy E. (2005): *Institutional Ethnography. A Sociology for People.* Oxford.

Solinger, Rickie (1993): "A Complete Disaster": Abortion and Politics of Hospital Abortion Committees, 1950–1970. *Feminist Studies,* 19 (2): 240–268.

Spradley, James P. (1980): *Participant Observation.* New York.

Steinkamp, Norbert; Gordijn, Bert (2003): *Ethik in der Klinik – Ein Arbeitsbuch. Zwischen Leitbild und Stationsalltag.* Neuwied, Köln, München.

Stemmer, Renate (2003): Zum Verhältnis von professioneller Pflege und pflegerischer Sorge. In: Deutsche Gesellschaft für Pflegewissenschaft e.V. (ed.): *Pflege und Gesellschaft. Sonderausgabe. Das Originäre der Pflege entdecken. Pflege beschreiben, erfassen, begrenzen.* Frankfurt am Main.

Steppe, Hilde (1991): Nursing in the Third Reich. *History of Nursing Journal,* 3 (4): 21–37.

Steppe, Hilde (1996): *Krankenpflege im Nationalsozialismus.* Frankfurt am Main.

Steppe, Hilde; Ulmer, Eva-Maria (1999): *"Ich war von jeher mit Leib und Seele gerne Pflegerin."* Über die Beteiligung von Krankenschwestern an den "Euthanasie"-Aktionen in Meseritz-Oberwalde. Frankfurt am Main.

Stevens, Tina M. L. (2000): *Bioethics in America. Origins and cultural politics.* Baltimore, London.

Storch, Janet L.; Griener, Glenn G. (1992): "Ethics Committees in Canadian Hospitals: Report of the 1990 Pilot Study". *Healthcare Management Forum,* 5 (1): 19–26.

Storch, Janet L.; Rodney, Patricia; Starzomski, Rosalie (2004): *Toward a moral horizon. Nursing Ethics for Leadership and Practice.* Toronto.

Storch, Janet. L.; Rodney, Patricia; Pauly, B.; Brown, Helen; Starzomski, Rosalie (2002): Listening to Nurses' Moral Voices: Building a Quality Health Care Environment. *CJNL,* 15 (4): November / December: 7–16.

Sweeney, Robert H. (1987): "Past, Present, and Future of Hospital Ethics Committees". *Delaware Medical Journal,* 59 (3): 183.

Taylor, Carol R. (1997): Everyday Nursing Concerns: Unique? Trivial? Or Essential to Healthcare Ethics? *HEC Forum,* 9 (1): 68–84.

Teel, Karen (1975): "The Physician's Dilemma: A Doctor's View: What the Law Should Be". *Baylor Law Review,* 27: 6–9.

Tewes, Renate (2002): *Pflegerische Verantwortung.* Bern.

Thomasma, David C. (1994): Toward a New Medical Ethics. Implications for Ethics in Nursing. In: Benner, P. (ed.): *Interpretative Phenomenology. Embodiment, Caring, and Ethics in Health and Illness.* Newbury Park, CA: 85–97.

Thompson, Joyce B.; Thompson, Henry O. (1985): *Bioethical decision making for nurses.* Norwalk, Connecticut.

Tong, Rosemarie (1997): *Feminist Approaches to Bioethics. Theoretical Reflections and Practical Applications.* Boulder, Colorado.

Toulmin, Stephen (1981): The tyranny of principles. *The Hastings Center Report,* 11 (6): 31–39.

Tronto, Joan (1994): *Moral Boundaries. A Political Argument for an Ethics of Care.* London.

Tronto, Joan (2001): Does Managing Professionals Affect Professional Ethics? Competence, Autonomy, and Care. In: DesAutels, Peggy; Waugh, Joanne (ed.): *Feminists Doing Ethics.* Lanham: 187–202.

Tronto, Joan (2006): Vicious Circles of Privatized Caring. In: Hamington, Maurice; Miller, Dorothy C. (ed.): *Socializing Care.* Lanham: 3–27.

Tulsky, James A.; Fox, Ellen (1996): Evaluating Ethics Consultation: Framing the Questions. *The Journal of Clinical Ethics,* 7 (2): 109–115.

Varcoe, Colleen et al. (2004): Ethical practice in nursing: working the in-betweens. *Journal of Advanced Nursing,* 45 (3): 316–325.

Varcoe, Colleen; Rodney, Patricia; McCormick, Janice (2003): Health Care Relationships in Context: An Analysis of Three Ethnographies. *Qualitative Health Research,* 13 (7): 957–973.

Veatch, Robert M. (1971): Experimental Pregnancy. *Hastings Center Report,* 1 (June): 2–3.

Veatch, Robert M. (1977): Hospital Ethics Committees: Is there a role? *Hastings Center Report,* 7: 22–25.

Veatch, Robert M. (1981): *A theory of medical ethics.* New York.

Veatch, Robert M. (1984): Autonomy's Temporary Triumph. *Hastings Center Report,* 14 (5): 38–40.

Vezeau, Toni M. (1992): Caring: From Philosophical Concerns to Practice. *The Journal of Clinical Ethics,* 3 (1): 18–20.

Vollmann, Jochen (2002): Klinische Ethikkomitees: Zur aktuellen Entwicklung in deutschen Krankenhäusern. In: Kolb, Stefan et al. (Hg): *Medizin und Gewissen. Wenn Würde ein Wert würde... Eine Dokumentation über den internationalen IPPNW-Kongress Erlangen 24. – 27. Mai 2001.* Frankfurt am Main: 277–287.

Vollmann, Jochen (2006): Ethik in der klinischen Medizin – Bestandsaufnahme und Ausblick. *Ethik in der Medizin,* 18: 348–352.

Vollmann, Jochen; Burchardi, Nicole; Weidtmann, Axel (2004): Klinische Ethikkomitees an deutschen Universitätskliniken – Eine Befragung aller Ärztlichen Direktoren und Pflegedirektoren. *Deutsche Medizinische Wochenzeitschrift:* 1237–1242.

Vollmann, Jochen; Wernstedt, Thela (2005): Das Erlanger klinische Ethikkomitee. Organisationsethik an einem deutschen Universitätsklinikum. *Ethik in der Medizin,* (17): 44–51.

Walker, Margaret Urban (1993): Keeping Moral Space Open. Images of Ethics Consulting. *Hastings Center Report,* March – April: 33–40.

Walker, Margaret Urban (1998): *Moral Understandings. A Feminist Study in Ethics.* New York.

Walker, Margaret Urban (2001): Seeing Power in Morality: A Proposal for Feminist Naturalism in Ethics. In: DesAutels, Peggy; Waugh, Joanne (ed.): *Feminists Doing Ethics.* Lanham: 3–14.

Walker, Margaret Urban (2003): *Moral Contexts.* Lanham, Boulder, New York, Toronto, Oxford.

Walker, Margaret Urban (2006): The Curious Case of Care and Restorative Justice in the U.S. Context. In: Hamington, Maurice; Miller, Dorothy C. (ed.): *Socializing Care.* Lanham, Boulder, New York, Toronto, Oxford: 145–162.

Walker, Robert M. et al. (1991): Physicians' and Nurses' Perceptions of Ethics Problems on General Medical Services. *Journal of General Internal Medicine,* 6 (September / October): 423–429.

Warelow, Philip J. (1996): Is caring the ethical ideal? *Journal of Advanced Nursing,* (24): 655–661.

Warren, Virginia L. (1992): Feminist Directions in Medical Ethics. In: Bequaert Holmes, Helen; Purdy, Laura M. (1992): *Feminist Perspectives in Medical Ethics.* Bloomington, Indianapolis: 32–45.

Watson, Jean (1985): *Nursing: Human science and human care. A theory of nursing.* 1st edition. Norwalk.

Watson, Jean (1988): *Nursing: Human science and human care. A theory of nursing.* 2nd edition. Norwalk.

Watson, Jean (1990): Caring knowledge and informed moral passion. *Advances in Nursing Science,* 13 (1): 15–24.

Watson, Jean (1996): *Pflege-Wissenschaft und menschliche Zuwendung.* Norwalk, Connecticut.

Watson, Jean (1999): *Post-modern Nursing and Beyond.* New York.

Watson, Jean (2001): Theory of human caring. In: Parker, M.E. (ed.): *Nursing theories and nursing practice.* Philadelphia.

Webster, G.C.; Baylis, Francoise E. (2000): Moral Residue. In Rubin, Susan B.; Zoloth, Laurie (ed.): *Margin of error: The ethics of mistakes in the practice of medicine:* 217–230.

Wehkamp, Karl-Heinz (2004): Die Ethik der Heilberufe und die Herausforderungen der Ökonomie. *Berliner Medizinische Schriften,* Heft 49. Berlin.

Weidner, Frank (1995): *Professionelle Pflegepraxis und Gesundheitsförderung. Eine empirische Untersuchung über Voraussetzungen und Perspektiven des beruflichen Handelns in der Krankenpflege.* Frankfurt am Main.

Welie, Jos V.M. (1998): Clinical Ethics: Theory or Practice? *Theoretical Medicine and Bioethics,* 19: 295–312.

Weir, Robert F. (1977) (ed.): *Ethical issues in death and dying.* New York.

Wiesing, Urban (2006): Ethikberatung in der klinischen Medizin: Stellungnahme der Zentralen Ethikkommission zur Wahrung ethischer Grundsätze in der Medizin und ihren Grenzgebieten (Zentrale Ethikkommission). *Deutsches Ärzteblatt,* 103 (24): A 1703–1707.

Wettreck, Rainer (2001): *"Am Bett ist alles anders" – Perspektiven professioneller Pflegeethik.* Münster.

Winslade, William J.; Ross, Judith W. (1986): *Choosing Life or Death. A Guide for Patients, Families, and Professionals.* New York.

Woll-Schumacher, Irene (1984): Sterben in Würde – ein Ergebnis sozialer Geborgenheit. *Universitas,* 39: 915–925.

Wolpe, Paul R. (1998): The Triumph of Autonomy in American Bioethics: A Sociological View. In: DeVries, Raymond; Subedi, Janardan: *Bioethics and Society. Constructing the Ethical Enterprise:* 38–57.

Yarling, Roland B.; McElmurry, Beverly J. (1986): The moral foundation of nursing. *Advances in Nursing Science,* 8 (2): 63–73.

Youngner, Stuart J. Jackson D.L., Coulton, C. et al (1983): A national survey of hospital ethics committees 'In Deciding to Forego Life-Sustaining Treatment'. *Report of the President's Commission for the Study of Ethical Problems in Medicine and Biomedical and Behavioral Research.* Washington, DC: 443–449.

Zink, Margo R.; Titus, Linda (1994): Nursing Ethics Committees – Where are they? *Nursing Management,* 25 (6): 70–76.

Zussman, Robert (1992): *Intensive Care: Medical ethics and medical profession.* Chicago.

Zussmann, Robert (2000): The Contributions of Sociology to Medical Ethics. *Hastings Center Report,* 30 (1): 7–11.